DISCOVER ... OF HEAL... INFORMATION!

Learn all about:

- BINGE EATING—how to control it
- ALAR—the carcinogen that produces larger, firmer, redder apples with a longer shelf life—and poisonous effects
- ALFALFA SPROUTS—the "health food" that can be harmful
- ARTIFICIAL COLORS—what they are, where they're found
- BODY FRAME—how to determine yours by elbow breadth
- VITAMIN SUPPLEMENTS—effects and side effects
- BOTTLED WATER—the sodium content of most popular brands
- COCOA, SHARP CHEESE AND PEANUTS as dental helpers
- DRUG AND FOOD interaction
- FEVER BLISTERS AND COLD SORES—a simple treatment
- DIABETIC EXCHANGE LISTS
- HERBS AND HERB TEAS that can be dangerous
- SALT SUBSTITUTES—a recipe you can make at home

Annette Natow, Ph.D., R.D. and Jo-Ann Heslin, M.A., R.D., are the authors of *No-Nonsense Nutrition for Your Baby's First Year, Geriatric Nutrition, Nutrition for the Prime of Your Life, No-Nonsense Nutrition for Kids, Nutritional Care of the Older Adult,* and *Megadoses; Vitamins as Drugs.* The authors have also held editorial positions at the *Journal of Nutrition for the Elderly, American Baby Magazine,* and *Prevention Magazine.*

Books by Annette Natow, Ph.D., R.D. and Jo-Ann Heslin, M.A., R.D.

Megadoses
No-Nonsense Nutrition for Kids
The Pocket Encyclopedia of Nutrition

Published by POCKET BOOKS

Most Pocket Books are available at special quantity discounts for bulk purchases for sales promotions, premiums or fund raising. Special books or book excerpts can also be created to fit specific needs.

For details write the office of the Vice President of Special Markets, Pocket Books, 1230 Avenue of the Americas, New York, New York 10020.

The Pocket
ENCYCLOPEDIA
of
NUTRITION

Annette B. Natow, Ph.D., R.D.
Jo-Ann Heslin, M.A., R.D.

PUBLISHED BY POCKET BOOKS NEW YORK

An *Original* publication of POCKET BOOKS

POCKET BOOKS, a division of Simon & Schuster, Inc.
1230 Avenue of the Americas, New York, N.Y. 10020

ISBN: 0-671-61278-6

First Pocket Books printing November, 1986

10 9 8 7 6 5 4 3 2 1

POCKET and colophon are registered trademarks
of Simon & Schuster, Inc.

Printed in the U.S.A.

To our families—Harry, Allen, Irene, Laura, Marty, George, Steven, Joseph, Kristen, and Karen—who help us through each project.

"We have come to the realization that nutrition is science rather than a bundle of old wives' rules; that foods, though so numerous and so varied in form, can be reduced to rather simple terms."

MARY SWARTZ ROSE, Ph.D.
Feeding the Family, 1919

CONTENTS

F

G

A

ACCENT is a trade name for the flavor enhancer MSG (monosodium glutamate).

See MSG

ACCUTANE (isotretinoin) is a derivative of vitamin A used to treat severe acne and psoriasis. Because of the danger of side effects it is used only for cases that cannot be helped in any other way. Persons on Accutane therapy should consult their physician before taking any vitamin supplements. Pregnant women should not use this medication.

ACEROLA CHERRY is also called Barbados-Cherry. These bright red fruits are the richest natural source of vitamin C. An 8 ounce glass of acerola juice contains 3,872 mg of vitamin C, almost forty times the amount in orange juice. You aren't likely to be drinking pure acerola juice since it normally is sold diluted as a fruit drink. It is most often found in vitamin C pills along with *bioflavonoids*.

ACETYLCHOLINE is a neurotransmitter produced in the brain. It carries nerve impulses (messages) from one nerve to another nerve or muscle. Memory depends on the level of acetylcholine in the brain. The amount of acetylcholine produced can be increased by taking in more choline or lecithin. This approach has been used to treat tardive dyskinesia (uncontrolled movements of face and upper body) which occurs after long-term use of antipsychotic drugs. It is also being investigated to treat memory disorders in the elderly.

See Lecithin

ACHLORHYDRIA is a lack of hydrochloric acid in the stomach juices. This condition occurs in many people over age sixty and can be a result of iron deficiency. Digestion and absorption of food and nutrients is affected and stomach bacteria may increase causing indigestion.

ACID is a substance that has a pH of 6.9 or lower. The lower the pH the more acid the food. The sour taste of vinegar, lemons, tomatoes and soft drinks is due to the acid in them.

pH Levels

Empty stomach	2.0
Lemons	2.2
Cola	2.3
Coffee	2.8
Sauerkraut	3.6
Tomatoes	4.2
Bananas	4.6
Budweiser beer	4.8
Potatoes	6.1
Milk	6.6
Shrimp	6.9

ACIDOPHOLUS MILK (Sweet Acidopholus Milk)
Milk cultured with lactobacillus acidophilus and other
bacteria. The sweet form now available tastes almost
the same as regular low-fat milk. It introduces friendly
bacteria into the intestine which help protect you from
harmful bacteria that can cause infections. Recent
studies show that the same L. acidophilus bacteria in
acidopholus milk can absorb fats and lower cholesterol
levels.

ADDITIVES Substances added to foods to preserve
them, improve taste or textures, add flavor, color or
nutrients. We eat about 150 pounds of additives a year,
with sugar and salt accounting for 140 pounds. The
other 10 pounds include gelatins, vitamins, minerals,
gums, etc.

See Artificial colors, Flavoring agents, GRAS, Natural
food colors, Preservatives, Processing agents

AD LIB (ad libitum) A common abbreviation meaning to take food as needed or as desired.

AFLATOXINS are a family of mold produced toxins
(mycotoxins or mold poisons) which can cause serious
poisoning. Aflatoxin B_1, the most potent, is toxic, carcinogenic (cancer-causing), mutagenic (changes gene
structure) and teratogenic (causes birth defects). Corn,
peanuts, rice, cottonseeds and nuts can be contaminated, usually due to high moisture levels during
storage. Aflatoxin levels in food are regulated by gov-
ernmental agencies and may not exceed fifty parts per
billion.

ALAR (Daminozide) is the most commonly used
pesticide and growth regulator in the apple growing
industry. It is used to grow larger, redder, firmer apples

with a longer shelf life. It is used primarily on Delicious, McIntosh and Stayman apples. Alar is absorbed into the fruit and cannot be removed by washing or peeling. It is believed to be a carcinogen but has not yet been banned. Residues of Alar, about one part per million, have been found in apple juice, apple sauce (baby and adult forms), peanuts, Concord grape juice and cherry filling. When exposed to heat or acids during processing, Alar is converted into a more dangerous carcinogen, UDMH (unsymmetrical dimethylhydrazine). The Environmental Protection Agency (EPA) has estimated that infants and children are at greater risk than adults because they eat more apple products. The EPA has postponed making a final decision on the use of Alar until 1988 when safety testing will be completed. In the meantime, a reduction in the amount sprayed on crops and lowered permissible residues will be instituted.

ALCOHOL comes in various forms such as methyl (wood alcohol) and isopropyl (rubbing alcohol). Ethyl alcohol or ethanol is the kind of alcohol we drink. Hard liquors like vodka, gin and rye are about 40 to 50 percent alcohol, wines are 10 to 14 percent alcohol and beers contain about 2 to 4 percent.

Alcohol does not need to be digested; it is simply absorbed from the digestive tract. It is a central nervous system depressant that can initially impair judgment, coordination, walking and speech. Emotions, memory and reflexes are affected next. Drunkenness and stupor will follow if drinking is continued.

Alcohol is a source of calories; 1 gram of alcohol equals 7 Calories.

See Alcohol in blood, Proof

ALCOHOL IN BLOOD Blood alcohol levels of 0.10 to 0.20 percent will cause most people to be intoxi-

Calories in Alcoholic Drinks

Drink	Size	Calories
Ale	1 mug (12 ounces)	150
Apricot brandy	1 cordial glass (1 ounce)	88
Beer	1 mug (12 ounces)	150
Beer, light	1 mug (12 ounces)	90
Brandy	1 cordial glass (1 ounce)	73
Creme de menthe	1 cordial glass (1 ounce)	96
Daiquiri	1 cocktail (3½ ounces)	124
Gin, Rum, Vodka, Rye (80 proof)	1 jigger (1½ ounces)	107
Gin, Rum, Vodka, Rye (100 proof)	1 jigger (1½ ounces)	132
Martini	1 cocktail (3½ ounces)	143
Scotch	1 jigger (1½ ounces)	102
Whiskey Sour	1 cocktail (3½ ounces)	138
Wine		
Champagne	1 wineglass (4 ounces)	84
Rose	1 wineglass (4 ounces)	81
Sherry	1 sherry glass (3 ounces)	120
Table	1 wineglass (4 ounces)	100

cated. Over 0.20 percent most people have trouble standing up or staying awake. Your blood alcohol level depends on many things such as:

Number of drinks
Type of drink
How fast you were drinking
If you drank on an empty stomach
Your body weight
Regular drinking habits
Emotional state
General physical health

See Proof

ALFALFA (Lucerne) tablets and capsules are often used to treat arthritis, reduce cholesterol, help diabetes, stimulate the appetite and act as a tonic. There is no scientific evidence to support these claims, although moderate use of alfalfa is safe and will provide some nutrients.

Alfalfa sprouts are available in supermarkets and salad bars. They are crunchy and refreshing but when eaten to excess they can be harmful. Toxic substances, called *saponins,* found in sprouts can damage red blood cells.

One cup of alfalfa sprouts contains:

> 23 Calories
> 2.9 g protein
> .8 mg iron
> 16 mg calcium
> 9 mg vitamin C

ALLERGY, *see* Food allergy

ALUMINUM is used to make cooking pots and utensils, antacids, baking powders, food additives and underarm deodorants. High brain levels of aluminum are found in persons suffering from Alzheimer's Disease and from "dialysis dementia," a condition seen in some patients on kidney dialysis. The significance of this elevated aluminum is not known. Aluminum, the most common element on earth, has not been shown to be essential for human health.

ALZHEIMER'S DISEASE is a progressive, common form of dementia in people over forty-five. There is forgetfulness, reduced ability to do simple calculations, and disorientation. Niacin and choline, both B vitamins, have been used to treat the condition with varying success. Niacin may help stimulate blood flow to the brain, while choline supplements given in the early stages of the disease slow its progress.

AMARANTH was called the "grain of the gods" by the Aztecs because they believed it prolonged life and vitality. Amaranth is good quality protein because it contains lysine, the amino acid or building block of protein that is lacking in most grains. Amaranth is also high in calcium. It is being promoted as a potential major cereal crop by the Rodale Research Center in Emmaus, Pennsylvania, who acts as a major seed source for amaranth.

Amaranth is also the original name for FD&C Red No. 2, a red food color that has been banned for use in foods, drugs and cosmetics.

AMINO ACIDS are the building blocks of protein. There are twenty-two different amino acids, nine of which are called essential. That description means that the nine essential amino acids must be obtained from the food we eat. The other thirteen amino acids can be made in the body.

Amino Acids

Essential	Nonessential
Histidine	Alanine
Isoleucine	Arginine
Leucine	Asparagine
Lysine	Aspartic Acid
Methionine	Cysteine
Phenylalanine	Cystine
Threonine	Glutamic Acid
Tryptophan	Glutamine
Valine	Glycine
	Hydroxyproline
	Proline
	Serine
	Tyrosine

Individual amino acids like lysine, arginine and tryptophan are frequently sold as supplements. Routine supplementation with amino acids is unnecessary for most healthy people but may be warranted in some situations.

See Protein, Protein complementation, Tryptophan

AMYGDALIN is a cyanide containing compound found in peach, apricot, apple, plum and bitter almond pits and is the main constituent of the controversial anticancer drug Laetrile. It is an extremely poisonous substance. Each gram of amygdalin is converted to approximately 60 mg of cyanide in the human body. This is a fatal dose for an adult.

See Laetrile

ANECDOTAL REPORTS are merely observations of an individual's experience. For example, a woman reported in a popular magazine that she improved her memory by drinking warm milk. This might call for further investigation but surely is not proof that warm milk can affect memory. Read testimonials cautiously and think of them as evidence that should be considered, tempered with a good dose of common sense.

See Double blind study

ANEMIA refers to a decrease in quantity or quality of red blood cells reducing body's oxygen supply. Pale skin and mucous membranes, weakness, fatigue, dizziness, shortness of breath, sore tongue, tingling in hands and feet all may be symptoms of anemia. The main causes are loss of blood through menstruation or hemorrhages, increased destruction or decreased production of red blood cells, and production of abnormal red blood cells. Some anemias are due to nutritional factors.

The following is a list of nutritional anemias:

Iron deficiency anemia Reduced size and number of red blood cells. Treated with iron supplements.

Hemolytic anemia Red blood cells easily damaged. Treated with vitamin E. Avoid iron supplements.

Megaloblastic anemia Enlarged red cells, reduced number. Treated with folic acid after ruling out possibility of pernicious anemia.

Pernicious anemia Enlarged red cells, reduced number. Treated with vitamin B_{12}.

Siderotic anemia Small, light colored red blood cells. Treated with vitamin B_6 (pyridoxine); may also have nonnutritive causes.

See Hematocrit, Hemoglobin, Pica

ANOREXIA NERVOSA is self-starvation with a weight loss of at least 25 percent of body weight. Ninety percent of the cases are young girls who start the abnormal eating behavior during adolescence. A typical anorexic is intelligent, introverted, sensitive, compulsive and a perfectionist. The disorder is not seen in underdeveloped countries. In addition to excess weight loss there is often a distorted body image in that a severely emaciated body is perceived as still being overweight. Loss of menstrual periods, vigorous activity, intolerance to cold, dehydration and soft hair growth over the body are other symptoms. Anorexics may also be bulimics, gorging on large quantities of food and then purging by excess laxative use or by vomiting. Mortality rate is about 10 percent, often due to mineral imbalance or toxic effects of emetics like syrup of ipecac.

See Bulimia

ANTACIDS are basic substances that neutralize stomach acid. Many people use them to relieve indigestion and its symptoms—gas, heartburn, pain, burning and nausea—because they believe they are caused by excessive acid. Actually, the normal condition of the stomach is very acidic, even more so than vinegar. In spite of this some people get relief from antacids and they have been shown to speed up the healing of ulcers. They are best taken one hour after meals when their effect will last three to four hours. If taken on an empty stomach they neutralize acid for only thirty minutes.

Some problems can develop when antacids are used for a long time. Most antacids contain sodium and should not be used by persons on a low sodium diet. Antacids also reduce iron absorption, so iron supplements should not be taken within two to three hours of antacid use. Calcium carbonate products *(TUMS)* can cause nausea and constipation if taken in excess. Magnesium is often added to counteract the constipating effect. These products also may cause a rebound of high stomach acidity several hours after use. Excess use of aluminum hydroxide containing antacids—Di-Gel, Maalox, Mylanta and Gelusil—will block phosphorus absorption leading to a loss of calcium. Long-term use can contribute to bone disorders like osteomalacia and osteoporosis.

Baking soda (sodium bicarbonate) is easily absorbed so it should never be used in high doses (more than 4 teaspoons) a day as it could cause alkalosis, a disturbance in acid-base balance in the body, and stomach rupture.

See Gas, Heartburn

ANTIOXIDANTS prevent or delay the breakdown of other substances by oxygen. They retard deterioration, rancidity and discoloration. Vitamins C and E are natural antioxidants. Many food additives act as antioxidants.

Common Antioxidants

Alpha tocopherol (vitamin E)
Ascorbic acid (vitamin C)
Sodium erythorbate (vitamin C derivative)
BHA (butylated hydroxyanisole)
BHT (butylated hydroxytoluene)
Sodium citrate
Propyl gallate
EDTA (ethylenediaminetetraacetic acid)

APHRODISIACS are food or other substances used to increase sexual desire. Licorice root, garlic, asparagus, caviar, lobster, truffles, ginseng and oysters (Casanova ate fifty raw oysters daily) have all been promoted as sexual stimulants. There is, however, no scientific basis for the use of any of these substances.

APOENZYME is the protein part of an enzyme.

See Enzymes

APPETITE, or the desire for food, is a learned response that is influenced by past experiences. It can be triggered by many different clues—time of day, smelling, hearing or seeing food, advertisements for food and talking about food. It is not the same as hunger, which is a physiological need for food.

APPLE CIDER VINEGAR, *see* Vinegar

ARSENIC is best known as a poison but has been used over the years as a tonic and as an aphrodisiac. Under the name *Salvarson,* an arsenic derivative was used to treat syphilis. Skin cancers may develop in persons who have been treated with arsenic years after exposure.

Fish, both finfish and shellfish, cereals, meats and salt are dietary sources of arsenic. We generally take in from 0.2 to 1.0 mg a day. Arsenic is given to pigs and poultry to promote growth and some laboratory animals seem to require arsenic for good health. Whether or not humans need arsenic has not yet been established.

ARTERIOSCLEROSIS refers to a group of diseases in which there is a thickening and loss of elasticity of the wall of the arteries. *Atherosclerosis* is a type of arteriosclerosis in which a yellowish plaque, made up of fat, blood, blood products, carbohydrate, calcium and fibrous tissue, is deposited inside the artery wall. This can reduce or cut off blood flow—leading to a heart attack or stroke.

See Heart attack

ARTHRITIS, or joint inflammation, is a general term for over 100 different ailments. *Osteoarthritis,* the most common kind, develops because of wear and tear on the joints, caused by overuse, stress and injury. *Rheumatoid arthritis* is an autoimmune disorder; the body's immune system turns on itself. This is more serious than osteoarthritis and can lead to crippling. *Gout* is another type of arthritis that can be considered a birth defect even though it doesn't show until adulthood.

See Gout, Nightshade vegetables, Osteoarthritis

ARTIFICIAL COLORS are used as coloring agents by manufacturers to make food more appealing. They make up 90 percent of all the colors used; natural colors are used for the remaining 10 percent of foods colored. Synthetic or artificial colors are more stable than natural food colors, resisting breakdown in air, light, heat or by interaction with food components. Food colors are listed on labels by means of their FD&C (Food, Drug and Cosmetic) number. The following table lists the limited group of certified food colors currently in unrestricted use.

See Natural food colors, FD&C approved food colors

Artificial Colors

Color	used in
Red No. 3	cherries in fruit cocktail
	candy
	baked goods
Red No. 40	soft drinks
	candy
	gelatin desserts
	pastry
	pet food
	sausages
Blue No. 1	baked goods
	beverages
	candy
Blue No. 2	pet food
	beverages
	candy
Yellow No. 5	gelatin dessert
Egg shade	candy
	pet food
	baked goods
Yellow No. 6	beverages
	sausage
	baked goods
	candy
	gelatin
Green No. 3	candy
	beverages

ARTIFICIAL SWEETENERS are also called non-nutritive sweeteners and provide a sweet taste with few or no Calories. These products are useful for diabetics but not as helpful for persons who want to lose weight.

Research shows that people who routinely use artificial sweeteners take in more calories in a day than those who use sugar.

Saccharin has been in use for over eighty years. It is 300 times as sweet as sugar but leaves a bitter aftertaste. It has been found to be a weak carcinogen (cancer-causing), and products containing it must have a warning label. In November 1985, the American Medical Association concluded that use of saccharin is not associated with increased risk of bladder cancer.

Cyclamates thirty times as sweet as sugar are currently banned in the United States because they were reported to be carcinogenic. The manufacturer is appealing this ban.

Aspartame (Equal, NutraSweet) is 200 times as sweet as sugar. It is made up of two amino acids (phenylalanine and aspartic acid) and has a small amount of Calories. It has no bitter aftertaste but cannot be used in cooking as heat breaks it down. There have been some reports of negative side effects such as seizures, headaches and changes in blood chemicals. People with the genetic disorder phenylketonuria (PKU) should not use aspartame. A warning label to this effect appears on products containing this sweetener. Many authorities suggest limited use by children and pregnant women.

See Diet foods, Diet sodas

ASCORBIC ACID is the chemical name for vitamin C.

See Vitamin C

ASPARTAME, *see* Artificial sweeteners

ATHEROSCLEROSIS, *see* Arteriosclerosis

ATHLETES, *see* Sports nutrition

B

BABY FOODS refer to foods other than breast milk,
formula or milk that are fed to infants during the first
year of life. These foods could be homemade or commercially prepared. Gerber, Beechnut and Heinz are
the major baby food manufacturers in the United
States; Milupa is a smaller manufacturer.

Commercially prepared infant food dates back to the
1920s, when pabulum and a few specialty items were
marketed for babies and sick adults. In 1928, Gerber
Products Company offered its first line of baby foods—
carrots, peas, prunes, spinach and vegetable soup—
sold in cans. Today, commercially prepared baby foods
are sold in jars, bottles, boxes and cardboard canisters.
A mother can choose items cooked, pureed and jarred
or dehydrated.

No matter what brand or type of baby food purchased the parent is assured that all foods are whole-
some and nutritious. Manufacturers have gone to great
lengths to produce quality baby food in keeping with
the latest developments in infant nutrition. No baby
food on the market today contains salt; many products

are unsweetened or have a very small percentage of sugar added; no chemical preservatives, artificial colors or flavorings are added; and the number of products containing starch thickeners has been reduced.

All ingredients are declared on the label, so it is easy to pick out the most nutritious items. Commercial baby foods offer fruits, vegetables, meats, cereal, combination foods, desserts and dinners. They are prepared strained, junior (thicker) and chunky to meet the developmental needs of the growing infant. All products available are convenient, safe and moderately priced. Jarred items are capped with a tamper-resistant lid. When opened, the center of the lid, normally depressed, pops up and a "pop" sound is heard. This assures the parent that the product has never been opened and the contents are safe.

BEAN CURD, or **tofu,** is made from soy milk the same way cheese is made from milk. It is sold as a white block about three inches square. Bean curd is a highly nutritious food. Cholesterol-free, it is a low-calorie, good protein food. It is bland and absorbs the flavors of foods it is cooked with.

Tofu Block-6 oz.

86 Calories
9.4 gm protein
5 gm fat
2.3 mg iron
150 mg calcium
8 mg sodium
trace vitamins

See Soybean

BEE POLLEN is considered an ergogenic (energy-boosting) food; it is used as an energy supplement by athletes. Pollen is the male sexual element of seed plants. It corresponds to sperm cells in humans. Containing more than 25 percent protein, 15 percent fat and over 50 percent carbohydrate, pollen is rich in B vitamins and iron. Its composition is similar to dried peas and beans but contains larger amounts of calcium and magnesium.

Critics have said that the boost athletes claim they get from bee pollen is purely psychological; in other words, bee pollen is merely a placebo. Another criticism is that because of the usual way the pollen is gathered, it contains fragments of bees and other debris that may cause allergic reactions in some users.

BEHAVIOR MODIFICATION techniques are used to treat eating problems like obesity, bulimia and anorexia nervosa. The concept is that eating behavior is learned and that bad eating practices can be unlearned. For treating obesity, keeping a diary of the type and amount of food eaten as well as time, place, emotional state, degree of hunger, and activities done while eating (such as reading or telephoning) can help detect problem areas. By means of contracts involving rewards and penalties, people try to control factors that stimulate poor eating behavior. Eating in one room only or eating more slowly are some techniques taught to help change eating patterns. Behavior modification based on rewards for eating has sometimes been used effectively with persons who have anorexia nervosa and to limit time during eating binges for bulimics.

BENZOPYRENES are carcinogenic substances made in farm soil by bacteria. They are also formed when meat is charcoal-broiled and this is considered to be the largest source of benzopyrene in food. It is formed when charcoal burns and the smoke deposits on the meat, when fat drips on the coals and vaporizes, or when the flames touch the meat. Placing a pan or aluminum foil between the meat and the charcoal smoke and flames substantially reduces benzopyrene levels. Cooking meat in frying pans and griddles also produces benzopyrenes. Cooking in a broiler with the heat source above the meat eliminates the formation of this carcinogen.

See Carcinogen

BERI-BERI is a nutritional deficiency disease caused by eating foods very low in vitamin B_1 (thiamin). The disease is found in populations that eat little else besides highly refined white flour, white rice or cassava. Chronic alcohol abuse can also cause beri-beri because alcohol, while containing no thiamin, uses up the body's supply of the vitamin and increases its excretion. Symptoms can include nerve and heart disorders, and fluid accumulation, causing swelling (edema). The disease can be cured with thiamin supplements.

BETACAROTENES are yellow pigments found in some deep yellow vegetables and fruits and dark green leafy and stem vegetables. Not every yellow fruit or vegetable is a good sources of betacarotene—for example, corn, pears and summer squash get some of their color from other pigments. Good sources are apricots, peaches, cantaloupe, carrots, sweet potatoes, winter squash (acorn, butternut), collards, spinach, asparagus and broccoli. Carotene is converted to vitamin A in the body. Research shows that eating foods rich in betacarotene may protect against certain types of cancer. A good source of this pigment should be eaten every day.

See Carotenemia

BEZOARS, *see* Intestinal impactions

BINGE EATING, simply defined, is a time when you eat to excess. In some people, this can be a sign of a serious eating disorder (bulimia); in others, it is simply a reaction to stress or a celebration. Most authorities feel binge eating is triggered by emotions that a person has trouble dealing with directly. All people binge sometimes. Normal-weight people who do it occasionally don't give the episode a second thought. Overweight people who binge usually feel guilty, which can lead to more eating.

There are specific steps that can be taken to help bring these episodes of overeating under control.

AT THE BEGINNING OF THE BINGE:

When you think a binge is starting, pause and remember *you are always in control.* You may choose to get away from the food, call a friend or plunge into an activity or even eat an acceptable substitute. Or you may choose to binge. Even when you are eating a whole cake, *you are in charge.* You are choosing to take each and every bite.

DURING THE BINGE:

Pause. Take a deep breath. Exactly *what are you feeling?* Is it hunger? Is it loneliness, sadness, anger or joy? *What do you really want?* Is it food? Or is it nurturing, a release, a high?

AFTER THE BINGE:

Forgive yourself immediately. Nobody is perfect. Everyone binges sometimes. Accept the binge and go right back to eating moderately. Fasting after a binge just starts the cycle of stuffing and starving. Vomiting or using laxatives upsets your body chemistry. After a binge *go back to eating normally.*

See Bulimia, Anorexia nervosa

BIO- is a prefix denoting life.

BIOFLAVONOIDS, formerly known as vitamin P, are natural pigments found along with vitamin C in fruits, vegetables, grains and flowers. They are often sold as supplements combined with vitamin C. Although bioflavonoids may be needed for lower forms of life, there is no established need for them in humans. They have been used, along with more conventional treatments, to treat bleeding disorders including heavy menstrual flow and bleeding gums, bruises and frostbite. More research is needed to determine their value for these disorders. Common cold sores (fever blisters) often respond to treatment with 200 mg of vitamin C plus 200 mg of bioflavonoids taken three times a day for three days started when the blister begins to erupt. At this time bioflavonoids have no known nutritional function and should not be considered essential nutrients.

BIOTIN, *see* Vitamins

BLACKSTRAP MOLASSES is a strongly flavored product, usually used for sweetening, made from sugar cane. It is richer in minerals than lighter colored molasses but because of its strong taste, only small amounts are used.

One tablespoon of blackstrap molasses contains:

> 116 mg calcium
> 2.3 mg iron
> 1 mg copper
> 43 Calories

BLAND DIETS have been recommended in the past for ulcers and other digestive disorders. Today they are not commonly used and have been replaced by more liberal individualized diets. Small, frequent meals, low in fat, with adequate protein and carbohydrate are used. Initially this diet plan eliminates fried foods, seasonings, colas, coffee and tea, which are added back to the diet as tolerated. Only alcohol, black pepper and meat extracts (bouillon) are not allowed.

BLOOD PRESSURE refers to the pressure or force of blood against the blood vessel wall. It is measured as millimeters of mercury and reported as two numbers written like this:

$$\frac{120}{80}$$

The upper figure, or systolic pressure, is the maximum pressure when the heart contracts and forces the blood through the arteries. The lower figure, or diastolic pressure, is the minimum pressure when the heart relaxes between beats.

The normal range of blood pressure is approximately:

$$\frac{100}{60} \text{ to } \frac{120}{80}$$

See Hypertension

BLOOD SUGAR, or blood glucose, is approximately 60 to 120 mg/dl (*see* p. 176) after a person has not eaten for eight hours. After age fifty, blood sugar levels go up about 1 percent a year. Fasting blood glucose levels can be increased by mental, emotional or physical stress. Because of this, levels are not considered abnormal unless they are more than 140 mg/dl.

High blood glucose levels are called hyperglycemia; low blood glucose levels are hypoglycemia.

See Diabetes, Glucose tolerance test, Hyperglycemia, Hypoglycemia.

BODY FRAME sizes, designated as small, medium and large, are used on Metropolitan Life Insurance Height-Weight Tables as a factor in determining appropriate weight for height. Instructions are provided for finding frame size by measuring elbow bones. It is difficult to do this accurately and it is possibly meaningless as well because there is no scientific basis for the concept of body frame size.

See Height-weight tables

How to Determine your Body Frame by Elbow Breadth

To make a simple approximation of your frame size:

Extend your arm and bend the forearm upwards at a 90 degree angle. Keep the fingers straight and turn the inside of your wrist away from the body. Place the thumb and index finger of your other hand on the two prominent bones on *either side* of your elbow. Measure the space between your fingers against a ruler or a tape measure.* Compare the measurements on the following tables.

These tables list the elbow measurements for medium-framed men and women of various heights. Measurements lower than those listed indicate you have a small frame and higher measurements indicate a large frame.

MEN

Height in 1" heels	Elbow Breadth
5'2" –5'3"	2½"–2⅞"
5'4" –5'7"	2⅝"–2⅞"
5'8" –5'11"	2¾"–3"
6'0" –6'3"	2¾"–3⅛"
6'4"	2⅞"–3¼"

---

*For the most accurate measurement, have your physician measure your elbow breadth with a caliper.

WOMEN

Height in 1" heels	*Elbow Breadth*
4'10"–4'11"	2¼"–2½"
5'0" –5'3"	2¼"–2½"
5'4" –5'7"	2⅜"–2⅝"
5'8" –5'11"	2⅜"–2⅝"
6'0"	2½"–2¾"

BODY TEMPERATURE is 98.6 degrees Fahrenheit.

See Fever, Temperature

BONE MEAL is ground animal bone used as a mineral supplement. It should not be used for this purpose as some samples have been shown to have undesirably high levels of lead. The Food and Drug Administration has recommended that bone meal supplements not be used by children and pregnant women.

See Calcium supplements.

BOTTLED WATER is becoming increasingly popular as a beverage. There is a great variation among available products. Some are obtained from a single, protected spring like Perrier while others may have many sources such as wells, rivers or the local water tap. Seltzer is tap water that has been filtered and carbonated. Club soda has added minerals and may have additives as well.

SODIUM CONTENT OF BOTTLED WATERS—8 OUNCES

Canada Dry Club Soda	44.00 mg
Deer Park	.39 mg
Evian	1.18 mg
Mountain Valley	.65 mg
Perrier	3.04 mg
Poland Spring	.32 mg
San Pellerino	10.02 mg
Vichy (Celestins)	277.40 mg
Club Soda (average)	60.00 mg

Brands sold in the state where they are bottled are not subject to federal purity regulations, so there is no assurance that they are free from contamination. Sodium levels vary also and some may be high in minerals, particularly in club soda where mineral salts (calcium and magnesium) are added to improve the taste.

See Perrier

BRAN is the outer coat of grain such as wheat, oats, corn and rice. It is high in fiber. One tablespoon of wheat bran has 7 Calories, .5 gm protein, 4 gm dietary fiber and tiny amounts of vitamins and minerals.

See Fiber

BREAST DISEASE, *see* Cancer, Fibrocystic breast disease

BREAST FEEDING is becoming popular once again in the United States. During the 1960s fewer than 15 percent of infants in this country were breast-fed. At the present time more than one half of infants leaving the hospital are breast-fed. Ninety-nine percent of all women can breast-feed; exceptions are those with severe anemia, heart disease, tuberculosis or kidney disease. When a breast feeding mother becomes pregnant, she should discontinue breast-feeding by the sixth month of pregnancy. Although babies may be adequately nourished with artificial formulas, breast-feeding has the advantage of providing the right combination of nutrients, providing immune bodies to protect the body against certain diseases and is mutually satisfying to mother and baby. It is also uncontaminated, readily available at the right temperature, least likely to provoke an allergy, easily digested and inexpensive.

During the first six months of life breast milk provides most of the nutrients the baby needs. Most authorities recommend an injection of vitamin K right after birth and some suggest supplements of vitamin D, iron and fluoride. The latter recommendation is controversial.

BREAST MILK, or human milk, is composed of 3.8 percent fat, 3.2 percent protein, 4.8 percent carbohydrates, 7 percent minerals and 87.5 percent water. In addition, breast milk contains other substances such as vitamins and immune properties that help protect the newborn from infection. Human milk, like cow's milk, provides 20 Calories an ounce, but is lower in protein and minerals, making it more ideal and better suited to the growth rate of infants.

See Breast feeding

BREWER'S YEAST (Saccharomyces) is a by-product of beer and ale brewing. It is used as a nutritional supplement because it is a rich source of B vitamins and when irradiated (*see* pg. 150) also contains vitamin D. It also contains protein—3.9 gm of protein in one tablespoon. One tablespoon of yeast provides about 28 Calories.

"Nutritional" or "food" yeast contains vitamin B_{12} because it is grown on a vitamin B_{12} enriched culture. It is one of the few nonanimal sources of this vitamin.

Mineral content of yeast depends on the source as yeasts can be grown on molasses, whey, wood pulp and other substances. Some may contain selenium or chromium while others do not.

Some people develop excessive, embarrassing gas when they take a yeast supplement. While some users adjust to the supplement, others will need to decrease their intake.

BULIMIA is also known as "gorge and purge syndrome." The person usually is female, has an abnormally increased appetite and can eat 10,000 to 20,000 Calories a day. Some women have been reported to eat $50 worth of food at a single time, including gallons of ice cream, whole bags of cookies and whole loaves of bread. This binge eating is followed by self-induced vomiting and/or use of large doses of laxatives and diuretics. Weight is normal to slim so that the condition often goes unnoticed. It has been estimated that 20 percent or more of female college students are bulimic. Dangers include serious tooth decay (which is caused by the acidic vomit), tears in the lower esophagus (food tube), difficulty swallowing and mineral imbalances.

See Anorexia nervosa

C

CAFFEINE, chemically a methylxanthine, is a stimulant found in coffee, tea, soft drinks, cocoa, chocolate and more than one thousand over-the-counter medications. Although it is not addictive, it is habit-forming and the body comes to depend on it. Many people can't get going without their "wake-up" cup of coffee. Caffeine is rapidly absorbed from the digestive tract and enters body tissues and organs within minutes. A "lift" is experienced within a half hour and can last for over three hours. The brain and heart are stimulated, increasing the capacity for mental and physical work. Urination is increased, as caffeine acts as a diuretic. Stomach acid secretion is increased as are levels of sugar and free fatty acids in the blood.

Man has used caffeine-containing plants for centuries and today every culture has a caffeine-containing food or beverage as a diet staple.

Caffeine acts like a drug in the body. Two hundred milligrams of caffeine (the amount in less than two cups of coffee) is a pharmacologically active dose. Some of its adverse effects are disturbed sleep, anxiety, irritability, heartburn and stomach upsets. Recent studies have associated caffeine use with fibrocystic breast disease and epithelial ovarian cancer and elevated serum cholesterol levels. Reports of effects of caffeine on blood pressure levels are contradictory.

Excess use of caffeine—the equivalent of four or more cups of coffee a day—can lead to dependency, with withdrawal symptoms of headache, nausea, vomiting and irritability when caffeine consumption is reduced.

Excess caffeine consumption in pregnancy is associated with smaller babies and greater risk of miscar-

Caffeine Content of Beverages and Foods

	Milligrams Average	Caffeine Range
Coffee (5-ounce cup)		
Brewed, drip method	115	60–180
Brewed, percolator	80	40–170
Instant	65	30–120
Decaffeinated, brewed	3	2–5
Decaffeinated, instant	2	1–5
Tea (5-ounce cup)		
Brewed, major U.S. brand	40	20–90
Brewed, imported brands	60	25–110
Instant	30	25–50
Iced (12 ounce glass)	70	67–76
Cocoa beverage (5-ounce cup)	4	2–20
Chocolate milk beverage (8 ounce)	5	2–7
Milk chocolate (1 ounce)	6	1–15
Dark chocolate, semi-sweet (1 ounce)	20	5–35
Baker's chocolate (1 ounce)	26	26
Chocolate flavored syrup (1 ounce)	1	4

Source: Food and Drug Administration, Food Additive Chemistry Evaluation Branch, based on evaluation of existing literature on caffeine levels.

riage. Intake of caffeine containing products should be reduced to no more than three daily. Caffeine can aggravate existing heart rhythm problems and should be avoided by persons with arrythmias.

Caffeine Content of Soft Drinks

Brand	Milligrams Caffeine (12-ounce serving)
Sugar Free Mr. PIBB	58.8
Mountain Dew	54.0
Mello Yello	52.8
TAB	46.8
Coca-Cola	45.6
Diet Coke	45.6
Shasta Cola	44.4
Shasta Cherry Cola	44.4
Shasta Diet Cola	44.4
Mr. PIBB	40.8
Dr Pepper	39.6
Sugar-Free Dr Pepper	39.6
Big Red	38.4
Sugar-Free Big Red	38.4
Pepsi Cola	38.4
Aspen	36.0
Diet Pepsi	36.0
Pepsi Light	36.0
RC Cola	36.0
Diet Rite	36.0
Kick	31.2
Canada Dry Jamaica Cola	30.0
Canada Dry Diet Cola	1.2

Source: Institute of Food Technologists (IFT), April 1983. Based on data from National Soft Drink Association, Washington D.C. IFT also reports that there are at least sixty-eight flavors and varieties of soft drinks produced by twelve leading bottlers that have no caffeine.

Caffeine Content of Drugs

Prescription Drugs	Milligrams caffeine per tablet/ capsule
Cafergot (for migraine headache)	100
Fiorinal (for tension headache)	40
Soma Compound (pain relief, muscle relaxant)	32
Darvon Compound (pain relief)	32.4

Nonprescription Drugs	
Weight-Control Aids	
Dex-A-Diet II	200
Dexatrim, Dexatrim Extra Strength	200
Dietac capsule	200
Maximum Strength Appedrine	100
Prolamine	140
Alertness Tablets	
Nodoz	100
Vivarin	200
Analgesic Pain Relief	
Anacin, Maximum Strength Anacin	32
Excedrin	65
Midol	32.4
Vanquish	33
Diuretics	
Aqua-Ban	100
Maximum Strength Aqua-Ban Plus	200
Permathene H_2O Off	200
Cold/Allergy Remedies	
Coryban-D capsule	30
Triaminicin tablets	30

Nonprescription Drugs	Milligrams caffeine per tablet/ capsule
Dristan Decongestant tablets and Dristan A-F Decongestant tablets	16.2
Duradyne-Forte	30

Source: FDA's National Center for Drugs and Biologics

Use of caffeine before an athletic event may be beneficial as it increases use of fatty acids for energy conserving the body's supply of glycogen. The diuretic action of caffeine may pose a problem for some athletes.

See Decaffeinated coffee, Methylxanthines

CALCIFEROL, *see* vitamin D.

CALCITRIOL (Rocaltrol) is the active form of vitamin D_1. Vitamin D taken in food or made in the skin is converted to its metabolically active form, a hormone, in the liver and kidneys. After this conversion vitamin D is called calcitriol.

See Vitamin D.

CALCIUM is an important mineral found in bones, teeth, blood and soft tissues. If you weigh 150 pounds, your body contains about three pounds of this mineral. Calcium has many functions: It builds bones and teeth; controls heartbeat; transmits nerve messages; is needed for muscle contraction and blood clotting; and activates many enzymes. If there is a deficiency of calcium, bones and teeth are not normal and growth is stunted. Studies show that low calcium intake during youth and early adulthood can contribute to the osteoporosis (adult bone loss) later in life. Recent research shows an association between calcium intake and high blood pressure in some people.

Adequate vitamin D is needed for calcium absorption; lactose (milk sugar), adequate protein, and an acid medium will increase calcium absorption as well. Excess fiber, fat and phosphorus or a vitamin D deficiency can reduce the amount of calcium absorbed. The efficiency of calcium absorption is reduced as we get older.

The recommended dietary allowance for calcium is 800 mg a day for adults, 1,200 mg a day for teens, pregnant and breast-feeding women. Some authorities believe that all women should increase their calcium intake to 1,200 mg to prevent or postpone bone loss.

See Calcium supplements, Minerals, Osteoporosis, Vitamin D

Calcium in Foods

Food	Portion	Milligrams of calcium
Almonds	12 nuts	38
Beef	3 ounces	10
Brazil nuts	4 nuts	28
Bread, white enriched	1 slice	24
Bread, whole-wheat	1 slice	24
Broccoli	½ cup	68
Butter	1 tablespoon	3
Cheese, American	1 ounce (1 slice)	195
Cheese, cheddar	1 ounce	204
Cheese, cottage, creamed	¼ cup	34
Cheese, cream	1 ounce	23
Cheese, mozzarella (whole milk)	1 ounce	163

Food	Portion	Milligrams of calcium
Cheese, Swiss	1 ounce	259
Collards	1 cup	357
Crackers, graham	2 crackers	10
Custard	½ cup	161
Egg	1 medium	28
Ice cream	½ cup	99
Margarine	1 pat	2
Milk, buttermilk	1 cup	296
Milk, nonfat dry (reconstituted)	1 cup	298
Milk, skim (1% fat)	1 cup	300
Milk, skim plus milk solids (protein fortified)	1 cup	349
Milk, whole	1 cup	291
Oatmeal, cooked	½ cup	11
Orange juice	1 cup	25
Peanuts, roasted without skin	1 tablespoon	5
Peas, cooked	½ cup	22
Perrier water	1 cup	32
Salmon	3 ounces	167
Sardines	3 ounces	372
Shrimp	3 ounces	98
Spinach	1 cup	51
Tofu	3 ounces	128
Tuna	3 ounces	7
Tums (antacid)	1 tablet	200
Turkey	3 ounces	7
Walnuts	¼ cup	41
Yogurt	1 cup	293

CALCIUM–PHOSPHORUS RATIO refers to the amount of calcium intake from the diet compared to phosphorus intake. Absorption of calcium is best when there is an equal amount of calcium and phosphorus or a 1:1 ratio or 1:1.5.

At the present time, most Americans take in much more phosphorus than calcium, so the ratio is about 1:4. This is due to high consumption of meat, soft drinks and some food additives.

Calcium: Phosphorus Ratio
Milk	1.3:1
Chicken breast	1:19
Flounder	1:16
Coca Cola	1:5.3
American cheese	0.8:1

CALCIUM SUPPLEMENTS have been recommended for those of us who get only the 450 to 550 mg of calcium a day that the typical American diet supplies. The Recommended Dietary Allowance for calcium is 800 mg for adults and many experts recommend even higher intakes—1,000 to 1,500 mg to help prevent adult bone loss (osteoporosis). There are indications from recent studies that adequate calcium intake may help prevent high blood pressure and also reduce the risk of colon cancer.

You can get all the calcium you need from food if you use plenty of milk and dairy products and green leafy vegetables. A quart of milk supplies over 1,000 mg of calcium along with other needed nutrients. If you do not eat enough of these foods, a supplement will help you make up the difference.

Common calcium supplements are calcium carbonate (ground oyster shells, limestone) calcium lactate, calcium gluconate and dicalcium phosphate. They come in tablets, capsules, powders or as liquids.

Calcium carbonate is 40 percent calcium, highest in percentage of calcium by weight; it is therefore the supplement of choice. It is available in some antacids—Tums, Alka Mints and Titralac; it is also available as ground oyster shells (Oscal, Oyster-Cal) or in synthetic forms (Cal-Sup, Chewable Biocal).

Calcium supplements may be combined with vitamin D added, to help use the calcium more efficiently. If you use these, don't take additional vitamin D in other supplements or you may take enough to be poisoned. Two thousand to five thousand IU of vitamin D a day is a dangerous level.

See Osteoporosis

CALCULI is the plural form of calculus. It refers to stones formed in passages or organs of the body when substances crystallize out of body fluids. Gallstones and kidney stones are common types of calculi.

See Kidney stones, Gallstones, Gout

CALORIC DENSITY refers to the number of Calories in a portion of food. Foods that contain a lot of fat like gravies, salad dressings, butter, margarine and oil have greater caloric density or more Calories. Foods that contain more carbohydrate or protein are not as high in Calories. Also, foods that contain a lot of water and/or fiber like most fruits and vegetables do, are not calorically dense foods.

CALORIES are a measure of the energy (heat) in food. Energy needed to do the body's work is measured as the amount of heat produced by the body's work. The energy value of food is measured in the Calories (more precisely kilocalories) that the food will produce when burned. The large Calorie (kilocalorie, kcal, C) is the amount of heat required to raise 1 kg of water 1°C.

We get Calories from carbohydrate, fat and protein in foods. One gram of carbohydrate or protein yields 4 Calories and one gram of fat 9 Calories.

See Joule

CANCER is a word with no precise medical meaning or definition. It is a general term used to stand for a large group of diseases involving malignant cells—carcinoma, sarcoma, melanoma, lymphoma, leukemias and others. A cancer cell comes from a normal cell that has lost control over its reproduction because of some initiating event. After the initiating event the body's immune response often destroys the mutated (changed) cells. At times, however, the immunological system does not protect and the cancer cells continue to grow and reproduce. At times the growth is slow and in other instances rapid.

Research suggests that diet affects more than half of all cancers in women and a third of all cancers in men. There appears to be three ways that food intake may initiate a cancerous growth.

Food may carry a *carcinogen*, like nitrites, into the body. A nutrient deficiency may favor cancer development. Trace mineral deficiencies and vitamin deficiencies have been linked to tumor growth in research reports. And last, nutrient excesses may alter body functioning and cause a malignant growth. All of the following have been linked to specific cancers:

EXCESSIVE INTAKE OF:	TYPE OF CANCER:
Whiskey or wine	lung
Beer	rectal
Refined foods	breast
Fats	breast, colon, rectal
Animal foods	colon, rectal, prostate
Calories	prostate
Smoked or pickled foods	esophagus, stomach

Based on what is currently known about nutrition and cancer, the best advice is to eat a wide variety of foods while keeping overall calorie intake low. The American Cancer Society, in 1984, issued these dietary guidelines "to help reduce the risk of getting cancer."

AMERICAN CANCER SOCIETY NUTRITION GUIDELINES

1. Avoid obesity.
2. Cut down on total fat intake.
3. Eat more high fiber foods, such as fruits, vegetables and whole grain cereals.
4. Include foods rich in vitamins A and C in the daily diet.
5. Include cruciferous vegetables such as cabbage, broccoli, brussels sprouts, kohlrabi, and cauliflower in the diet.
6. Be moderate in consumption of alcoholic beverages.
7. Be moderate in consumption of salt-cured, smoked and nitrite-cured foods.

See Aflatoxins, Beta carotene, Carcinogen, Cruciferous vegetables

CANDIDIASIS is a form of vaginitis caused by the common yeast *Candida albicans.* Some women have repeated bouts of this condition. A popular theory proposes that some of these sufferers have a whole body allergy to a toxin produced by Candida. A weakened immune system results along with other symptoms like headache, premenstrual tension, fatigue, depression and constipation. The theory of the "candidiasis syndrome" claims that it causes a craving for foods containing yeast and foods that will nourish the yeast. Suggested dietary treatment is avoiding yeast breads, aged cheese, vinegar, alcohol, mushrooms and practically all carbohydrates including sugar, flour and milk. Such a severely restricted diet can cause deficiencies and there is no scientific basis for its use. In fact the American Academy of Allergy and Immunology found "no published proof that *Candida albicans* is responsible for the syndrome" and that the concept is "speculative and unproven."

CANDY was first made in Venice in the middle of the

Calorie Content of Candies

Candy	Serving Size	Calories
Almond Joy	1.6 ounce	220
Baby Ruth	2.28 ounce	320
Bubblicious	one piece	25
Cadbury Almond	2.0 ounce	310
Chiclets	one piece	6
Hershey's Kiss	one	25
Jelly Beans	25	100
Joyva Halvah	1 ounce	160
Kit Kat	1.5 ounce	210
Lifesavers Fruit Flavors	1 piece	10
Milky Way Bar	2.1 ounce	270
Reese's Pieces	35 pieces	140
Snickers Bar	2.0	270
Whitman's Sample pieces— Vanilla Caramel	1	79

1400s. Today the United States is the leading candy manufacturer and Americans eat over seventeen pounds per person per year, with Life Savers as the top-selling candy. Over 2,000 different confections are made, all of which fall under the regulation of the U.S. Food and Drug Law which requires the use of pure ingredients and nonpoisonous flavorings and colorings. Candies always contain some type of sugar or syrup (even "sugarless" varieties have sugar substitutes or sugar alcohols as sweeteners) and may contain egg, fats, gelatin, gums, lecithin, milk or milk products, cooked starches, fruits, nuts and flavorings. Because of the high sugar and fat content of most varieties, candies should be saved for occasional treats.

CARAMEL COLOR is produced when sugar is heated to approximately 350°F (150°C). The brown sweet syrup is used for color and flavor in gravies, cookies, and other baked goods. It may be added to breads to give the rich appearance of whole wheat.

See Natural food colors

CARBOHYDRATE LOADING, see Glycogen loading

CARBOHYDRATES are one of the energy yielding nutrients we eat.

They provide the body with energy; the excess is stored as fat. Some carbohydrate is stored as glycogen in the liver and muscles. Carbohydrates include sugars, starch, cellulose and other fibers. The sugars and starches are digested and used in the body while cellulose and other fibers (gums, pectin, mucilages) cannot be digested.

Carbohydrates are classified according to the number of carbon atoms in their structures. Monosaccharides (single sugars) with 3,4,5 or 6 carbons are usually the building blocks of more complex carbohydrates. The five carbon sugar ribose is part of the nucleic acids DNA (deoxyribonucleic acid) and RNA (ribonucleic acid). Xylose is another 5 carbon sugar and is used in some chewing gums.

Six carbon sugars (monosaccharides) include fructose or fruit sugar, glucose, the sugar in our blood and galactose found in milk sugar.

Twelve carbon sugars (disaccharides) are made from two monosaccharides, and include lactose (milk sugar), maltose and sucrose which is table sugar. Table sugar can be made from sugar cane or from sugar beets. Most sweeteners that we use—corn syrup, honey, maple syrup—are combinations of mono- and disaccharides. Polysaccharides are large sugar complexes made up of many chains of monosaccharides. Most glucose is stored in plants as starch. Starch as it comes from plants is insoluble; when it is cooked, the starch granules swell as they absorb water, breaking the cell walls and becoming digestible. Cellulose, an indigestible carbohydrate, is the most common polysaccharide in nature and is a major source of fiber in the diet.

At least 100 grams of carbohydrate (400 Calories) is recommended daily.

See Glycogen, Sugar

CARCINOGEN is a cancer-causing substance which is man-made or naturally occurring in nature. Research has identified approximately thirty substances as carcinogens. Food often acts as the carrier, transporting a carcinogen into the body. Benzopyrene, nitrites, cyclamates, sassafras, DES (diethylstilbesterol), EDB (ethylene dibromide), PCBs (polychlorinated biphenyls) and saccharin have all been suspected of carcinogenicity. If the link between a chemical and cancer appears strong, the chemical must be removed from the food supply as mandated by the Delaney Clause of the Federal Food, Drug and Cosmetic Act. For example, sassafras was banned in 1958; cyclamates in 1970; and DES in 1979. Currently saccharin and EDB are under investigation and final action on their status in the food supply is pending.

See Benzopyrene, Cancer, Nitrosamines, Saccharin

CARIOGENIC refers to a food or food ingredient which promotes dental cavities (caries). Sticky sugars, like raisins or caramels, adhere to the teeth and are more likely to promote decay. Table sugar (sucrose) is one of the most cariogenic of foods.

See Dental health

CARNITINE is an amino acid made in the body that helps body cells turn fatty acids into energy. Carnitine is obtained from animal foods and wheat germ. A vegetarian diet is likely to be low. Carnitine has been recommended as a supplement for those with coronary artery disease but there is no proof that it is helpful for this.

CAROB (St. John's Bread), a plant pod, is the source of locust bean gum, used as a food additive to improve texture and thicken foods. The ground dried pod is used as a cocoa substitute. Carob is used by some people in preference to cocoa because it contains no stimulants while cocoa contains theobromine, a caffeinelike substance. It is naturally sweet, so it may eliminate the need for sugar in some recipes.

If you wish to substitute carob for cocoa in recipes, use about 1½ to 2 times as much carob as the amount of cocoa the recipe calls for. Carob and cocoa look alike but do not taste the same.

CAROTENE, *see* Betacarotene

CAROTENEMIA refers to a condition in which the palms of hands and soles of feet are yellowed, reflecting high blood levels of the yellow pigment carotene. Eating large amounts of deep yellow-orange fruits and vegetables and dark green leafy vegetables can cause this in some people. Usually the carotene in food is converted to colorless vitamin A but if more is eaten than can be converted, the excess carotene remains in the blood and colors the skin. This condition is harmless, and can be distinguished from jaundice, a symptom of liver disease, because in carotenemia the whites of the eye do not turn yellow.

CATARACTS are a clouding over of the lens of the eye. If the lens becomes completely opaque, there is vision loss. Rats fed diets deficient in vitamin B_2

(riboflavin) can develop cataracts along with other eye disorders. Burning, itching, tearing and development of extra blood vessels in the eye are associated with riboflavin deficiency in humans, but cataracts are not.

Some studies show a greater occurrence of cataracts in persons who continue to produce high levels of the enzyme lactose and consume large amounts of milk throughout their lives. More research is needed to determine if this association is significant and is an important factor in cataract formation.

See Lactose intolerance

CELIAC DISEASE (gluten sensitive enteropathy) refers to malabsorption due to a sensitivity to gluten, a protein found in wheat, rye, barley and oats. The allergy damages the lining of the small intestine, interfering with the absorption of fats and some sugars and starches.

Celiac disease begins in childhood and lasts throughout life. In adults it is called sprue. Affected children grow poorly, have frequent stools with high gas and fat content so the stool floats on water and is difficult to flush down the toilet.

A diet utilizing rice, corn and soy beans in place of gluten-containing grains is recommended. The child may also become temporarily sensitive to sugar and milk sugar (lactose) because of damage to the intestine. This disappears after a gluten restricted diet is followed. Nutrient supplements are used at the start of treatment, but after the intestinal lining heals and normal absorption is restored they may be discontinued.

CELLULITE is the name used for the lumpy fat deposits that dimple hips and thighs. It is claimed that this fat is different from regular fat in that it has to be broken up by massage or other methods before you can lose it, even when you diet.

In fact, fat is fat and there is no special type. Singling out some fat with a special name is simply a way for people to make money by offering unusual treatments to help get rid of it.

CEREALS, or grains, are the seeds from cereal plants which are members of the grass family. Wheat, oats, corn, barley, buckwheat, rice and rye are popular grains in the United States. Triticale, a hybrid of wheat and rye, is a new cereal variety. Today, Americans are eating fewer cereal/grain foods, about one half as much as in 1900. We get about 20 percent of our calories from grains, 19 percent of our protein, over 33 percent of iron and 42 percent of vitamin B_1 (thiamin), 28 percent of niacin (a B vitamin) and less than 2 percent of fat. Cereals/grains are a nutritious, filling, low-fat food.

Cereal Glossary

Bran: Outer layer which encases germ and endosperm; rich in fiber

Endosperm: Surrounds germ and is rich in starch

Enriched: Restores some important nutrients (the three B vitamins and iron) that have been removed in refining

Fortified: Adding one or more nutrients that were either not present at all or that were not present in large amounts; vitamin D fortification of cereal is common

Germ: The seed or innermost part of a cereal kernel; rich in nutrients

Refined: Bran or the germ or both have been removed

Whole grain: An entire cereal kernel which is ground, rolled or cracked

CHEESE is the solid part, or curd, found when milk is heated with a starter—usually the enzyme rennet—which begins the coagulation of the cheese curd. The liquid part, whey, is drained off. It can take ten or more pounds of milk to make one pound of cheese. Americans eat on the average over twenty-two pounds of cheese each year and the amount eaten increases yearly. In 1960 we ate less than nine pounds each. Cheese is a highly concentrated food, consisting mainly of protein and fat with little or no carbohydrate.

American Cheese (pasteurized, processed)—one ounce

107 Calories
6.5 gm protein
0.5 gm carbohydrate
8.4 gm fat
318 mg sodium
195 mg calcium

Creamed Cottage Cheese—1 ounce

30 Calories
3.8 gm protein
0.8 gm carbohydrate
1.2 gm fat
64 mg sodium
26 mg calcium

Brie—1 ounce

94 Calories
5.8 gm protein
0.1 gm carbohydrate
7.8 gm fat
176 mg sodium
52 mg calcium

Cheddar—1 ounce

112 Calories
7.0 gm protein
0.6 gm carbohydrate

Cheddar—1 ounce

9.1 gm fat
197 mg sodium
211 gm calcium

Swiss—1 ounce

104 Calories
7.7 gm protein
0.5 gm carbohydrate
7.8 gm fat
74 mg sodium
259 mg calcium

CHELATED MINERALS are minerals chemically bound to another substance, usually an amino acid. It is claimed that minerals in this form are more easily absorbed. Chelated minerals cost more but there is no evidence to support the claim of greater absorbability.

CHELATION involves the injection of substances into the body where they bind to metals like lead. The bound metal is then passed out in the urine. Penicillamine and EDTA (ethylemediaminetetraacetic acid) are common chelating agents. Chelation is helpful in the treatment of lead poisoning and excess iron accumulation. Its use has also been suggested to reduce the plaque in arteries. This treatment is questionable, expensive and may be harmful.

CHEWING is the mechanical action in the mouth that results in the breaking up and moistening of food to allow it to pass down into the digestive tract. Many food fads have grown up around a fascination with chewing. William Gladstone, Prime Minister of England in the nineteenth century, said he owed his success in life to the rule about chewing. "I have made it a rule to give every tooth of mine a chance and when I eat I chew every bite thirty-two times." This habit helped him lose weight.

An American entrepreneur, Horace Fletcher, was an unhappy five feet six inches and 217 pounds when he heard about Gladstone and started to diet by chewing each mouthful vigorously. He eventually lost sixty-five pounds. He became such an advocate of chewing that he developed "Fletcherism," which promoted the idea of chewing each mouthful forty to fifty times with the head hanging down toward the chest until the food became a liquid consistency. Upton Sinclair, a Fletcher convert, immortalized Fletcherism in a little ditty.

> "Nature will castigate
> Those who don't masticate."

In the September 1909 issue of the *Ladies' Home Journal*, "Fletcherism" was the lead article. Many other important magazines of the time also endorsed Fletcher as did universities of the day. Dartmouth gave him an honorary degree for outstanding accomplishments. More recently, Sattalaro's book, *Recalled by Life*, recommended chewing every mouthful 50 to 150 times which will give the eater a euphoric "high." The "high" from this diet more likely is a result of the ketotic effect (an accumulation of acidlike substances in the blood which disturbs the body's neutrality [pH balance]) of the limited food selection, which is mainly brown rice and a little green tea. Another explanation is that the repetitive chewing has a hypnotic effect.

CHICORY is a plant with edible leaves and roots. The root is roasted and ground and used as a coffee extender.

CHILDREN'S NUTRITION refers to the nutritional requirements of children from the age of one year through the end of their growth spurt in adolescence. A one-year-old child needs about 1,000 Calories a day; a three-year-old needs 300 to 500 Calories more. Appetite decreases markedly around age one as the child's growth rate slows. Thereafter, appetite will fluctuate, increasing during times of growth and decreasing when growth is less active. Often parents are concerned because, at times, it seems like the child is eating little or nothing, yet this seemingly starving child is full of energy and looks remarkably healthy. Often parents overestimate what a child needs daily, based on their own appetite and the amount they eat. The following four food groups were scaled down to reflect the needs of a younger child and serve as a useful daily guide in meal selection.

During adolescence, growth and appetite increase. The nutrients an adolescent needs are as much or more than an adult needs. For further information on the daily food needs during adolescence, *see* Four food groups.

Daily Food Guide for the Preschool Child (ages 2–5)

A preschool child needs daily:

Milk
  2 cups
  1 serving = ½ cup

Use whole milk, evaporated milk (reconstituted with water), skim milk, nonfat dry milk, buttermilk, cheese,* yogurt.

Meat, Fish, Poultry, and Protein-Rich Foods
  3 servings
  1 serving = 1 oz.

Eggs, cheese, dried peas or beans, tofu, peanut, or other nut butters may be substituted for a serving of meat, fish or poultry.

Vegetables and Fruit

 4 or more servings
 1 serving of vegetable = ¼ cup
 1 serving of fruit = 1 small fresh fruit
 = ¼ cup cooked or canned fruit

1 serving of a vitamin C-rich food (orange, grapefruit, melon, strawberries, broccoli, tomatoes, coleslaw). 1 serving of a vitamin A-rich food, dark green or deep yellow-orange in color (spinach, sweet potato, carrot, apricot and mango).
2 or more servings of other fruits and vegetables (including potatoes).

Bread, Cereal, Rice, Pasta

 3 to 4 servings
 1 serving = ½ slice bread
 = ¼ cup cooked cereal, pasta, or rice
 = ⅓–½ cup dry cereal

Use only whole grain and enriched products.

Daily Food Guide for the School-Age Child (Ages 6–10)

A school-age child needs daily:

Milk

 2 cups
 1 serving = 1 cup

Use whole milk, evaporated milk (reconstituted with water), skim milk, nonfat dry milk, buttermilk, cheese,* yogurt.

Meat, Fish, Poultry, and Protein-Rich Foods

 2 servings
 1 serving = 2 oz.

Eggs, cheese, dried peas or beans, tofu, peanut, and other nut butters may be substituted for a serving of meat, fish or poultry.

Vegetables and Fruits
  4 or more servings
  1 serving of vegetable = ⅓ cup
  1 serving of fruit   = 1 medium fresh fruit
                          = ⅓ cup cooked or canned fruit

1 serving of a vitamin C-rich food (orange, grapefruit, melon, strawberries, broccoli, tomatoes and coleslaw).
1 serving of a vitamin A-rich food, dark green or deep yellow-orange in color (spinach, sweet potato, carrot, apricot and mango).
2 or more servings of other fruits and vegetables (including potatoes).

Bread, Cereal, Rice, Pasta
  4 servings
  1 serving = 1 slice of bread
            = ½ cup cooked cereal, pasta, or rice
            = ½ cup dry cereal

Use only whole grain and enriched products.

Daily Food Guide for the Preteen (Ages 11–13)

A preteen needs daily:

Milk
  2–3 cups
  1 serving = 1 cup

Use whole milk, evaporated (reconstituted with water) milk, skim milk, nonfat dry milk, cheese,* yogurt.

Meat, Fish, Poultry, and Protein-Rich Foods
  3 servings
  1 serving = 2 oz.

Eggs, cheese,* dried peas or beans, tofu, peanut, and other nut butters may be substituted for a serving of meat, fish or poultry.

*1 ounce serving cheese = 1 cup milk

Vegetables and Fruits
    4 or more servings
    1 serving of vegetable = ½ cup
    1 serving of fruit   = 1 fresh fruit
                            = ½ cup cooked or canned fruit

1 serving of a vitamin C-rich food (orange, grapefruit, melon, strawberries, broccoli, tomatoes, and coleslaw).
1 serving of a vitamin A-rich food, dark green or deep yellow-orange in color (spinach, sweet potato, carrots, apricots and mango).
2 or more servings of other fruits and vegetables (including potatoes).

Bread, Cereal, Rice, Pasta
    4 or more servings
    1 serving = 1 slice bread
              = ½ cup cooked cereal, rice, or pasta
              = ½ cup dry cereal

Use only whole grain and enriched products.

CHINESE RESTAURANT SYNDROME refers to headache, neck and chest pain, palpitations and tightness across the chest—symptoms that are believed to be due to a sensitivity to monosodium glutamate (MSG). MSG is a flavor enhancer widely used in processed foods and in Chinese food. The symptoms, which can be provoked by as little as one teaspoon of MSG, begin within one hour after eating.

Recent research has linked vitamin B_6 (pyridoxine) deficiency and the Chinese Restaurant Syndrome.

See Flavoring agents, MSG

CHLORINE is an essential mineral in the body where it is found as the chloride ion. A large amount of the chloride is part of the stomach secretion hydrochloric acid. As such, it is necessary for digestion in the stomach and activation of enzymes. It also functions in maintaining the acid-base balance and water-electrolyte balance in the body.

The Recommended Dietary Allowance estimates a safe and adequate intake of chlorine to be 1,700 to 5,100 mg a day for adults. We can get all we need as part of sodium chloride (table salt).

See Minerals

CHOLECALCIFEROL is a chemical name for vitamin D.

See Vitamin D

CHOLELITHIASIS, *see* Gallstones

CHOLESTEROL is a fatlike alcohol that is found in every cell in the body. Cell membranes, brain tissue and the covering of nerves contain cholesterol. Bile acids, hormones, vitamins D and sebum, the fat that keeps your skin smooth, are made from cholesterol. You make about two-thirds of the cholesterol you use and get the other third from food.

All meats, milk, finfish, shellfish and chicken contain cholesterol. The major food source is egg yolk; an average yolk contains about 250 mg. Liver, heart, kidney and brains are other rich sources. There is no cholesterol in plant foods like corn oil, peanut butter, fruit, cereal or grains.

Over 100 years ago cholesterol was identified in the deposits (plaque) on artery walls. Since then research points to an association between blood levels of cholesterol and the development of coronary artery disease, heart attack and strokes.

Recently it has become evident that it is not simply

the blood level of cholesterol but the type or form of cholesterol that is important. Cholesterol is part of both high density lipoproteins (HDL) and low density lipoproteins (LDL). A high level of low density lipoproteins is a risk factor for heart disease while high levels of high density lipoproteins are protective.

See Heart attack, Hypercholesteroliemia, Lipoproteins

Cholesterol in Foods

Food	Portion	Milligrams of cholesterol	Calories
Margarine, vegetable oil	1 teaspoon	0	36
Bacon fat	1 tablespoon	1	126
Bread	1 slice	1	70
Milk, skim	1 cup	5	90
Sour cream	1 tablespoon	5	26
Cottage cheese, 1% fat	½ cup	5	81
Cream, half and half	1 tablespoon	6	20
Chicken fat	1 tablespoon	9	126
Mayonnaise	1 tablespoon	10	100
Yogurt, low fat, fruit flavor	1 cup	10	231
Butter	1 teaspoon	11	36
Lard	1 tablespoon	12	126
Butter, unsalted	1 teaspoon	13	45
Fish sticks, frozen	1 stick	15	40
Sardines, canned in oil	1 sardine	15	40
Cottage cheese, creamed	½ cup	17	130
Caviar	1 tablespoon	25	32
Swiss cheese	1 ounce	26	104
Ice cream	½ cup	27	165
American cheese	1 ounce	27	93
Cheddar cheese	1 ounce	30	112
Milk, regular whole	1 cup	34	168

Food	Portion	Milligrams of cholesterol	Calories
Cream cheese	2 tablespoons	34	99
Frankfurter	1	34	170
Cake, from mix with chocolate frosting	1 slice	36	175
Cinnamon roll	1	39	174
Salmon, broiled	3½ ounces	47	200
Clams	3½ ounces	50	52
Halibut, broiled	3½ ounces	60	214
Chicken, white meat	3 ounces	67	115
Beef	3 ounces	75	245
Chicken, dark meat	3 ounces	75	160
Veal, lean	3 ounces	85	210
Shrimp, fried	½ cup	120	225
Tuna, canned in oil	3½ ounces	125	197
Tuna, canned in water	3½ ounces	125	127
Shrimp, canned	3½ ounces	150	116
Egg	1 egg	252	78
Liver	3½ ounces	370	135
Chopped liver	3 ounces	735	210

CHOLINE is a substance which has an affinity for fat. It is a component of lecithin, which is used commercially as an emulsifier. Choline prevents the development of a fatty liver, an abnormal state where the liver loses its ability to function. Choline is used to treat alcoholic fatty liver.

Animal studies show that giving choline can increase the brain's neurotransmitter acetylcholine. It is useful for persons who have tardive dyskinesia (involuntary repetitive movements of the face) that develops after long-time use of antipsychotic drugs. Choline is also being studied for use in Alzheimer's Disease, a memory disorder in the aged.

Eggs, brewer's yeast, liver, wheat germ, soybeans, cabbage, wheat bran and beans are rich sources of choline. Choline can also be made in the body. It is often incorrectly referred to as a B vitamin, but it is not a vitamin, because it can be made in the body.

See Alzheimer's Disease, Acetylcholine, Lecithin, Neurotransmitters

CHROMIUM is a mineral and an essential part of the glucose tolerance factor (GTF). It increases the action of insulin, a hormone involved in glucose (sugar) metabolism. Chromium supplements can improve the body's ability to handle glucose but only if there is a deficiency of this mineral. Chromium supplements have also lowered serum cholesterol levels. The LDL cholesterol was reduced while HDL cholesterol increased. This is a positive change.

The Recommended Dietary Allowance estimated a safe and adequate daily intake of chromium to be 50 to 200 mcg for adults. Usual diets eaten in the United States may not supply this amount. Grains and cereals are good sources of chromium, as is brewer's yeast. The amount of chromium in the soil will affect the amount of mineral found in the foods grown in it. Cooking acid foods in stainless steel pots may leach out some of the chromium from the steel into the food.

See Cholesterol, Minerals

CITRUS FRUITS are juicy subtropical fruits, including all varieties of oranges, grapefruit, lemons and limes. These delicious fruits are low in calories and good sources of vitamin C, folic acid, bioflavonoids, potassium, pectin and fiber. One medium orange supplies 80 mg of vitamin C, more than the Recommended Daily Allowance for that vitamin along with 300 mg of potassium and 60 mcg of folic acid. Eating the whole fruit (minus the peel) is more beneficial than drinking the juice. The fiber, pectin and bioflavonoids are found mainly in the membranes and the peel of the fruit.

COBALAMIN is a chemical name for vitamin B_{12}.

See Vitamin B_{12}

COD LIVER OIL has been used for many years as a tonic. It is becoming popular now as a "natural" vitamin supplement. It is a good source of vitamins A and D and also has some vitamin E. Cod liver oil contains EPA and DHA, the fish oils that have been shown to offer some protection against heart disease. Even though cod liver oil is made from livers of cod and other similar fish, it should be considered as a supplement, not as a food; its high content of vitamin D could lead to poisoning if too much is taken. One tablespoon contains 30 mcg (1,200 IU) of vitamin D, 12,000 IU of vitamin A, 3 mg of vitamin E and 85 mg cholesterol.

See EPA

COFFEE is a mildly stimulating beverage with fewer than 5 Calories per cup (not including added sugar and cream) and small amounts of niacin, a B vitamin (1.2 mg per cup). Its consumption almost equals milk, the second most popular drink after soft drinks. The per capita consumption of coffee in the United States is over twenty-six gallons. Consumption has been decreasing since 1946.

Coffee is one of the most complex chemical mixtures used as a food and has been implicated as a causative agent in heart attacks, high blood pressure, pancreatic cancer, ulcers, low blood sugar, fetal abnormalities and fibrocystic breast disease. There is no conclusive evidence to support these claims at this time.

See Caffeine

COFFEE CREAMERS, or coffee whiteners, are non-dairy creamers; they do not contain cream although they are used as substitutes for it. They may contain vegetable fat (often palm oil or coconut oil), corn syrup, casein (milk protein) and coloring along with additives to emulsify and stabilize. One teaspoon of a typical powdered coffee creamer has 10 Calories and practically no other nutrients.

While powdered coffee creamers are useful when no refrigeration is available, they are not desirable for persons on a low cholesterol diet because they contain saturated fats.

There have been reports of children developing severe protein deficiency after they had been fed coffee creamers in place of milk. Coffee creamers are not nutritionally equal to milk.

COLORS, *see* Artificial colors, Natural food colors

COPPER is a mineral associated with iron in the body. It functions as part of enzymes in hemoglobin formation, and in cellular energy production. An adult's body contains approximately 100 to 150 mg of copper.

The estimated safe and adequate daily intake of copper is 2 to 3 mg. The average American diet provides this amount. Copper is found in many foods, particularly meat (liver), shellfish (oysters), nuts, seeds, dried peas and beans, and whole grains.

Whipping egg whites in copper bowls makes them frothier and more durable than when whipped in glass or china. Egg whites contain conalbumin, a protein that binds with copper and acts as a stabilizer.

See Minerals

CARRAGEENAN (Irish moss) is a mixture of non-digestible polysaccharides (fiber). It is used as a food additive to emulsify, stabilize and thicken. It is commonly used in milk products like chocolate milk, ice cream and in infant formula.

See Processing agents

CREATININE is a nitrogen-containing compound formed during breakdown of body tissue and excreted in the urine. Creatinine normally is formed in proportion to muscle mass and its excretion in the urine is related to the amount of muscle in the body. Reduced creatinine is found in malnourished people; increased creatinine may occur when there is kidney damage.

CREATININE COEFFICIENT IN PERSONS OF IDEAL BODY WEIGHT:

23 mg/kg ideal weight for men
18 mg/kg ideal weight for women

CRUCIFEROUS VEGETABLES are a family that includes broccoli, brussels sprouts, cabbage, cauliflower, rutabagas, turnips, kohlrabi and mustard. In animal experiments these foods have been shown to inhibit the growth of cancer cells. The American Cancer Society has recommended eating these foods regularly in their dietary guidelines for reducing the chance of getting many types of cancer.

See Cancer

CYANOCOBALAMIN is a chemical name for vitamin B_{12}.

See Vitamin B_{12}

CYCLAMATES, *see* Artificial sweeteners

D

DECAFFEINATED COFFEE is coffee from which the caffeine has been removed.

There are three major decaffeination processes. In the *standard process*, heated water is circulated over the coffee beans and then an organic solvent (methylene chloride) is used to extract the caffeine. The *direct contact method* uses a heavier organic solvent and no water. In the newer *Swiss water process* (also called Pure), warm water is circulated continuously over green coffee beans until no more than 3 percent of the caffeine remains. In this process the coffee retains more flavor. The U.S. Food and Drug Administration sets an official maximum of ten parts per million by weight in the green coffee beans for the residue of organic solvent.

Decaffeinated coffee is becoming more popular. In 1962 only 4 percent of coffee consumed was decaffeinated; in 1984, 22 percent was decaffeinated. Decaffeinated coffees contain only .8 to 8.4 mg caffeine per 6 ounce cup compared to 66 to 150 mg in 6 ounces of regular coffee. Decaffeinated coffees cost more because they go through extra processing and because less is sold.

DEHYDRATION refers to excessive water loss from the body. This can occur because of too little fluid intake or too large a fluid loss or both. A variety of situations can lead to insufficient fluid intake—for example, inability to manage the act of drinking, poor mental status, unavailability of liquids or absence of thirst. Prolonged vomiting, diarrhea, hemorrhage, excessive urination, diuretic use, prolonged fevers, burns, excess sweating, and seepage from wounds may all cause dehydration. This can lead to reduced blood volume, circulatory failure, reduced kidney function, decreased intestinal movement (peristalsis) and poor nutrient absorption. Minerals (electrolytes) are lost along with water, so these too must be replaced.

See Water, Diarrhea, Vomiting

DENTAL DISEASE refers to cavities (caries) and gum (periodontal) disease. In the U.S. we spend $12 to $14 billion a year on dental care. Six and a half billion alone is spent to fill cavities. Virtually all Americans have some decayed teeth by the time they become adults; the average 15-year-old has ten decayed, filled or missing teeth.

A cavity is a bacterial infection of the tooth. The infection starts when bacteria found in dental plaque ferment sugars we eat to form organic acids. These acids attack the tooth, eroding the enamel surface. If the acid attack is frequent enough, eventually the enamel is worn away and the bacteria enter the tooth resulting in a cavity or bacterial infection. Once damaged, tooth enamel cannot repair itself, therefore preventive dental care is very important.

To interrupt the bacteria→sugar→acid→cavity cycle, dietary habits can be altered so that sugar is less available to the oral bacteria. Everytime we eat a food containing sugar—even an apple—our teeth are bathed in acid for thirty minutes. It is more important *how many* times a day we eat sugar than how much sugar we eat at one time. It would be wiser to eat sweets along with a meal rather than have three sweet candies during the afternoon. Each time we eat that small piece of candy the thirty-minute cavity cycle is set in motion.

Recent dental research has begun to show that certain foods—peanuts, sharp cheeses and cocoa—have a cariostatic (decay-slowing) effect on teeth. These foods inhibit dental plaque formation so the bacteria cannot adhere to the tooth. Eating them at the end of a meal helps to neutralize the thirty minute acid attack.

See Fluoride, Fluoridation, Periodontal disease, Xylitol

DHA, *see* EPA

DIABETES (diabetes mellitus) refers to a condition where there are abnormally high levels of sugar (glucose) in the blood. When the sugar level reaches approximately 180 mg/dl, sugar is passed out in the urine. Insulin, a hormone made by the pancreas, is needed for the body to use glycose normally. The reason for the high sugar (glycose) level in the blood is that little or no insulin is produced or that the insulin produced is inactive. This inability to use glucose normally is called glucose intolerance.

There are two general types of diabetes. Insulin dependent diabetes mellitus (IDDM), formerly called Type I or juvenile diabetes, usually occurs before middle age. Symptoms may include excess thirst and urination, increased appetite along with weight loss and poor healing. Persons with this form of diabetes need to have daily insulin injections to compensate for their deficient supply of this hormone. Diet is controlled to balance the intake of calories and carbohydrate with the availability of the injected insulin.

Noninsulin dependent diabetes mellitus (NIDDM), formerly called Type II or maturity-onset diabetes, is the most common form of the disease. It occurs in persons middle-aged or older who, though often overweight, may be free of other symptoms. NIDDM may be controlled simply by weight loss, if needed, along with a balanced diet of regular meals and avoiding concentrated sweets. If dietary control is not sufficient to stabilize blood sugar levels, oral hypoglycemic drugs or insulin injections may be needed.

Persons who have close relatives with NIDDM would be wise to keep their weight normal, to avoid developing the disease which is believed to run in families.

See Diabetic food exchanges, Glucose tolerance test

DIABETIC FOOD EXCHANGES are lists of foods grouped together because they contain similar amounts of carbohydrates, fats, protein and therefore have similar Calories. There are six categories: Milk, bread, vegetables, fruit, meat and fats. Food in any one group can be substituted or exchanged for any other food within the same group. Similar systems of exchange lists are used for other kinds of diets like weight loss, salt restriction, fat restriction and others.

DIABETIC EXCHANGE LISTS

Milk Exchange:	80 Calories, 12 gm of carbohydrate, 8 gm of protein, trace of fat
	Example: 1 cup of skim milk
Bread Exchange:	70 Calories, 15 gm of carbohydrate, 2 gm protein
	Example: 1 slice of bread
Vegetable Exchange:	25 Calories, 5 gm of carbohydrate, 2 gm protein
	Example: ½ cup carrots

Fruit Exchange:	40 Calories, 10 gm of carbohydrate Example: 1 small apple (lean meat)
Meat Exchange:	55 Calories, 7 gm protein, 3 gm fat Example: 1 oz. chicken breast (Meats with more fat are listed separately, as fat and calorie levels are higher.)
Fat Exchange:	45 Calories, 5 gm fat Example: 1 teaspoon butter or margarine

DIARRHEA refers to frequent, watery bowel movements caused by infections, drugs, allergic or nervous reactions and also by some serious disorders. Excess intake of naturally sweet foods such as apple juice can lead to diarrhea as can "sugar-free" candy, cookies and chewing gum sweetened with sorbitol or mannitol. Even too much vitamin C can cause loose stools. In the past persons with diarrhea were given liquids but no food. It was believed that an empty stomach was helpful in controlling the condition. Now the recommendation is to eat whatever is desired except for fatty foods, which should be avoided until diarrhea stops. Apples, bananas, rice, cottage cheese and crackers are good choices.

In addition, Oral Rehydration Therapy (ORT) is given to counteract the loss of fluid and minerals due to passage of frequent, watery stools. Pedilyte, Lytren, Resol and Infalyte are available without a prescription. You can make a similar rehydration solution at home by combining:

    4   tablespoons sugar
    ½ teaspoon salt

¼ teaspoon salt substitute (potassium chloride sold
under various brand names such as:
Adolph's, Diamond or Morton)
½ teaspoon baking soda (bicarbonate of soda)
1 liter of water (1 quart and 2 tablespoons)

The water used should be clean. Hot water from the faucet can be used but not boiling water.

The mixture has also been used effectively for "traveler's diarrhea."

Most diarrhea is self-limiting. When the fluid balance becomes normal, the person usually recovers in a day or two. If diarrhea persists for more than 2 days, consult a doctor.

DIET refers to the foods that are usually eaten. Diets may be changed (modified) when there are certain health problems like high blood pressure or diabetes. In everyday language, diet means only one thing— eating in a different way to lose weight. At any time, at least 20 percent of all Americans (forty million people) are on some kind of weight loss diet. Every year or so a new wonder diet plan is published, "guaranteed" to help you lose weight and keep it off. They are almost always variations on the same theme. Following are some popular diet themes.

Few Foods: This type of diet is based primarily on a few foods which can be dangerous or at the least may result in nutrient deficiencies. It is usually so boring that people will not stick with it. Examples: Banana and Skim Milk diet, The Grapefruit diet, Lecithin B_6 Apple Cider Vinegar Kelp Diet, The Beverly Hills Diet.

High Fiber: Diet cannot be tolerated by many who find it to be irritating and gas producing. Very high fiber coupled with low calorie intake can result in mineral deficiencies. Examples: The F-Plan Diet, Pritikin Permanent Weight Loss Diet.

Low-Calorie: Diet may be so low in calories that nutrient deficiencies can develop if diet is used for a prolonged period. Usually allow limited choices of food. Examples: Richard Simmons Never Say Diet Diet, Pritikin Diet, Weight Watchers Quick Start.

Low Carbohydrate: Diet usually is high in protein and fat while supplying less carbohydrate than is advisable for optimum health. This diet plan may also be called high fat or high protein. It can cause rapid weight loss for a short time (one or two weeks), largely because of water loss. Ketosis, with loss of minerals, can result from inadequate carbohydrate for normal metabolism. Examples: Dr. Atkins Diet Revolution, Complete Scarsdale Diet, Stillman: The Doctor's Quick Weight Loss Diet.

Modified Fast: Diet utilizes very low calorie formulas; can be dangerous, as some deaths have occurred in persons following these very restricted diets. Examples: Dr. Linn's Last Chance Diet, The Cambridge Diet, Herbal-life

See Ketosis

DIETARY GUIDELINES for healthy Americans were first recommended by a committee of scientists from the U.S. Department of Agriculture and the Department of Health and Human Services in 1980. The guidelines were revised and reissued in 1985. The seven dietary guidelines suggested are intended for healty Americans who wish to modify their eating behavior to reduce the risk of chronic diseases such as premature heart disease, diabetes, high blood pressure, and high cholesterol. The guidelines emphasize variety, balance and moderation in the diet

1. Eat a variety of foods.
2. Maintain desirable weight.
3. Avoid too much fat, saturated fat and cholesterol.

4. Eat foods with adequate starch and fiber.
5. Avoid too much sugar.
6. Avoid too much sodium.
7. If you drink alcoholic beverages, do so in moderation.

The first two guidelines are the framework of a good diet and the next five guidelines describe special characteristics of a good diet. The guidelines do not recommend specific amounts of vitamins, minerals, fat, sugar, sodium, alcohol, starch or fiber. They do suggest, however, that the population as a whole should choose a diet that reduces calories from fats, sugars and alcohol while increasing calories from complex carbohydrates and increasing the intake of dietary fiber.

A complete explanation of the revised 1985 Dietary Guidelines is available to consumers in the booklet "Nutrition and Your Health, Dietary Guidelines for Americans" (Home and Garden Bulletin No. 232). To obtain a copy write to the Consumer Information Center, Pueblo, Colorado 81009.

DIET FOODS are foods sold for use by persons on low calorie diets. According to present regulations, the term diet foods must be used only for low-calorie or reduced calorie or for calorie-restriction-diet foods as they are defined by law.

See Restriction labeling, Low calorie foods, Lite or light foods

DIETHYLENE GLYCOL is a solvent used in antifreeze. On occasion it has been found as an adulterant in imported wine; it had been added to sweeten the wine. The wine was subsequently recalled because diethylene glycol is not an approved additive.

DIETITIAN refers to a person with a bachelor's or higher degree in nutrition and dietetics who plans and supervises the preparation of food and evaluates the nutritional well-being of those who eat it. Dietitans may or may not be registered. Registration, identified by the initials "R.D." (registered dietitian) after a name, indicates that the person has successfully completed training, has served a work apprenticeship and has passed a national registration exam. To maintain registration, continuing education is required. Some states license dietitians in addition to national registration. A dietitian is eligible for membership in the American Dietetic Association. Over half of the professionally trained dietitians work in health-care facilities but they may also work in research, education, public health, industry or commerical food service (restaurants, airlines and other types of food services).

See Nutritionist

DIET PILLS include amphetamine-type drugs (which since 1980 can no longer be prescribed for weight loss), fiber bulking agents, diuretics and some hormones. These are said to be aids to weight loss.

Amphetamine-type drugs depress the appetite, so that the dieter will eat less food. Their long-term effectiveness has been questioned as their appetite-depressing effects may last only a couple of weeks. As addiction, insomnia, dry mouth, hypertension, cardiac irregularities, impotence, constipation and allergy are some of the side effects, it is no wonder that the Food and Drug Administration (FDA) has banned these drugs for use in weight control. A related drug, phenylpropanolamine hydrochloride (PPA) is available in nonprescription diet pills.

Bulking agents, such as methyl cellulose, carrageenen and sodium alginate, are not digestable. They expand as they absorb water, filling the stomach; this slows down the passage of food and also makes a person feel full. Bulking agents may have a laxative effect and it is not certain if they help weight loss or not.

Thyroid hormones have been given to people who have normal thyroid function to help weight loss by speeding up metabolism. Use of these hormones is controversial because the weight that is lost is mainly muscle, not fat. However, some authorities believe that their stimulating effect on body metabolism may help compensate for the normal body response to a low calorie diet—lowered metabolic rate. The FDA has issued warnings about using thyroid hormones in weight reduction.

Two other hormones, human chorionic gonadatropin (HCG) and progesterone, have been found to be of little or no benefit for weight loss. The effectiveness of growth hormone is still being investigated.

See PPA

DIET SODAS are soft drinks that are sweetened by a noncaloric sweetener like saccharin or asparatame (NutraSweet). Labeling requirements for diet soft drinks requires listing the presence of sweeteners, both natural and artificial, as well as caffeine. Most authorities recommend avoiding heavy use of diet sodas, especially by children, pregnant and breast-feeding women.

See Caffeine, Soda

DIGESTION is both a mechanical and chemical process. The process begins in the mouth where food is masticated (chewed) by the teeth into smaller particles and wet by saliva. The food *bolus* passes through the esophagus into the stomach where further mixing takes place. The food, now called *chyme,* goes into the small intestine where it is hydrolyzed (digested) and absorbed out of the digestive tract and into the body. There are enzymes in the mouth, stomach and small intestines that aid in the breakdown of food, readying it for absorption into the body.

DIURETICS (water pills) are substances that increase the flow of urine. These medications are often used to treat high blood pressure. Thiazide-type diuretics (Hydrodiuril, Hygrotin) cause potassium loss from the body. Persons taking them are often advised to eat potassium-rich foods.

People mistakenly believe that some foods and vitamins act as natural diuretics. That is not true. Only alcohol, caffeine and water increase urine flow.

See Potassium

DMSO (Dimethylsulfoxide) is a veterinary drug that has been touted as a cure or benefit for arthritis. Its effectiveness in treating arthritis has not been established and it can have dangerous side effects—chemical burns and vision damage.

DOLOMITE is a mineral compound that contains calcium carbonate and magnesium carbonate. Dolomite tablets have been recommended as a good calcium supplement because they supply twice as much calcium as magnesium, which is close to the RDA ratio for these minerals. It is also claimed that the magnesium aids the absorption of calcium; however, this is not true. Magnesium is added to calcium supplements to counteract the constipating effects of the calcium, not to improve absorption. As dolomite is a natural compound found in the earth, its composition varies. There have been reports of lead poisoning resulting from use of dolomite that was contaminated with lead.

Some other dolomite samples have been contaminated with other toxic minerals—for example, arsenic, mercury and aluminum. The Food and Drug Administration has issued a warning that children and pregnant women should not use dolomite supplements.

See Calcium supplements.

DOUBLE BLIND EXPERIMENTS refers to studies in which neither the subjects nor the investigators know which subjects are controls and which are the experimental group until after the experiment is over.

Scientific information is often obtained by the use of controlled experiments. An example of this is where two groups of people similar to each other in terms of age, sex and health are selected. One group is considered experimental, the other is the control. Persons in the experimental group, for example, may be given vitamin C daily to see if it has any effect on the number of colds they develop. The control group is given a placebo (a non-active substance) instead of the vitamin and the number of colds each group develops is compared. In a doubleblind study the subjects would not know which group they were in and neither would the persons conducting the study. This is done to eliminate any bias such as expecting one group to do better than the other that could affect the study's results.

See Anecdotal reports

DRUG AND FOOD INTERACTION Drugs and foods can each affect your body's reaction to the other. Drugs can change your sense of taste and smell; change appetite; cause nausea and vomiting; decrease nutrient absorption; and displace nutrients in body reactions. Food can change the effectiveness of a drug. Some drugs and foods do not get along well together. Here are some common examples.

Drug	Effect on nutrition
Antacids	
Aluminum hydroxide (Maalox)	Decreases absorption of phosphate, vitamin A; inactivates thiamin; deficiency of calcium and vitamin D
Calcium carbonate (Tums, Titrilac)	Decreases absorption of fatty acids; nausea
Anticoagulant	
Coumarin (Coumadin)	Vitamin E enhances action; vitamin K reduces effectiveness, limit food high in vitamin K; limit alcohol, caffeine, green tea; silicon additives in cooking oils inhibit absorption
Anticonvulsants	
Barbiturates (phenobarbital)	Decreases absorption of vitamin B_{12} and thiamin; deficiency of folate, vitamins D and K
Hydantoin (Dilantin)	Decreases serum folate, pyridoxine, calcium, vitamin B_{12} and D; increases excretion of vitamin C; increases copper; do not take with foods enhanced with monosodium glutamate (MSG)
Antidepressants	
Tricyclic (Elavil)	Increases food intake (large amounts may suppress intake)
Monoamine oxidase inhibitors (Parnate, Nardil)	Interacts with tyramine in food causing headaches, hypertensive crises, diarrhea

Drug and Food Interactions *(cont.)*

Drug	Effect on nutrition
Anti-inflammatory Agents	
Colchicine	Decreases absorption of vitamin B_{12}, carotene, fat, lactose, sodium, potassium, protein, cholesterol
Glucocorticoids (Prednisone)	Decreases absorption of calcium and phosphorus; increases food intake and salt retention
Zomepirac (Zomax)	Nausea, anorexia, flatulence
Antihypertensives	
Hydralazine (Apresoline)	Anorexia, vomiting, nausea, diarrhea, constipation
Captopril (Capoten)	Decreases taste; anorexia, nausea, vomiting, diarrhea
Methyldopa (Aldomet)	Increases need for vitamin B_{12} and folate; diarrhea, constipation, nausea, vomiting, flatulence, dry mouth
Antimetabolites	
5-Fluorouracil (Efudex)	Diarrhea, altered taste, sore mouth; decreases protein absorption; increases need for thiamin
Methotrexate	Decreases absorption of vitamin B_{12} and folate; nausea, vomiting, diarrhea
Antimicrobials	
Ampicillin	Do not take with fruit juice; nausea, vomiting, diarrhea
Chloramphenicol	Increases need for riboflavin,

Drug and Food Interactions *(cont.)*

Drug	Effect on nutrition
	vitamin B_{12} and pyridoxine
Erythromycin (Erythrocin or E-Mycin)	Do not take with fruit juice; diarrhea, nausea, vomiting
Isoniazid (INH)	Decreases absorption of vitamin B_{12}; pyridoxine deficiency; secondary niacin deficiency; dry mouth
Lincomycin (Lincocin)	Diarrhea, nausea, vomiting
Methenamine (Mandelamine)	Maintain adequate fluid intake
Metronidazole (Flagyl)	Dry mouth, nausea, vomiting, unpleasant taste
Neomycin	Decreases absorption of fat, carotene, protein, vitamins A, D, K, B_{12}, potassium, sodium, calcium, iron
Nitrofurantoin (Furadantin)	Maintain adequate protein; nausea, vomiting, diarrhea
Sulfamethoxazole and trimethoprim (Septra, Bactrim)	Decreases absorption of folate; decreases bacterial synthesis of folate, vitamin K and B vitamins; increases urinary excretion of vitamin C
Sulfisoxazole (Gantrisin)	Decreases absorption of folate; decreases bacterial synthesis of folate, vitamin K and B vitamins; increases urinary excretion of vitamin C
Tetracycline	Nausea, vomiting, diarrhea; decreases absorption of fat, protein, calcium, iron, magnesium, zinc; decreases

Drug and Food Interactions *(cont.)*

Drug	Effect on nutrition
	bacterial synthesis of vitamin K; do not take with milk or foods high in iron
Antipyretics	
Acetaminophen (Tylenol)	Carbohydrates retard absorption
Acetylsalicylic acid (aspirin)	Decreases serum folate; increases excretion of vitamin C, thiamin, potassium, amino acids, glucose; nausea, gastritis
Indomethacin (Indocin)	Anorexia, nausea, vomiting, diarrhea, flatulence
Phenylbutazone (Butazolidin)	Decreases absorption of folate; increases excretion of protein; constipation, nausea, vomiting
Hypercholesterolemic Drug	
Cholestyramine (Questran, Cuemid)	Decreases absorption of fats, vitamins A, D, E, K, B_{12}, folate; constipation
Laxatives	
Bisocodyl (Dulcolax)	Do not take with milk since this may cause disintegration of the enteric coating
Dioctyl-sodium sulfosuccinate (Colace)	Take with milk or juice; increases absorption of cholesterol and vitamin A; alters absorption of water and electrolytes; nausea, vomiting, diarrhea, bitter taste
Mineral oil	Decreases absorption of vitamins A, D, E and K

Drug and Food Interactions *(cont.)*

Drug	Effect on nutrition
Phenolphthalein (Ex-Lax)	Decreases absorption of vitamins A, D, E and K
Miscellaneous	
Diazepam (Valium)	Constipation, nausea, salivary changes
Digitalis (Lanoxin, Digoxin)	Increases excretion of potassium, magnesium, calcium; nausea, vomiting, anorexia, diarrhea; incompatible with protein hydrolysates; *caution with herbal teas*
Griseofulvin (Fulvican)	Altered taste, dry mouth
Levodopa (Larodopa)	Anorexia, nausea, vomiting, dry mouth, constipation; increases need for vitamins B_{12}, C, pyridoxine; increases excretion of sodium, potassium; *limit foods rich in pyridoxine*
Levothyroxine sodium (Synthroid)	*Do not take with goitrogenic foods, i.e., brussels sprouts, cabbage, mustard greens, cauliflower, spinach, kale, rutabaga, soybeans, turnips*
Lithium carbonate (Lithane, Lithotabs, Lithonate)	*Not compatible with decreased salt diet*
Iron salts (Feosol, Fergon)	When taken with whole grains, absorption is decreased; when taken with vitamin C, absorption is increased

Drug and Food Interactions *(cont.)*

Drug	Effect on nutrition
Penicillamine	Loss of taste; increased requirement for pyridoxine; increased excretion of zinc, iron, copper, pyridoxine; anorexia, nausea, vomiting, diarrhea
Potassium chloride (K-Ciel, Kaochlor, K-Lor, K-Lyte-Cl, Slow-K)	Decreases absorption of vitamin B_{12}; diarrhea, nausea, vomiting
Cimetidine (Tagamet)	Bitter taste, diarrhea, constipation
Thiazide diuretics (Diuril, Hydrodiuril)	Increases excretion of sodium, potassium, chloride, magnesium, zinc, riboflavin; anorexia, nausea, vomiting, diarrhea, constipation

E

EDB, ethylene dibromide, used for many years as a gasoline additive, is a pesticide that had been used in soil, stored grains, in milling machinery and on some fruits since the 1940s. Its use was phased out in 1983 and 1984 because EDB was shown to be a carcinogen in animal tests. Critics of the ban say the risk from EDB was overestimated and that a person would have to eat 250,000 times as much food as normal to equal the cancer-causing dose given to laboratory animals. Irradiation can be used as a substitute for this chemical pesticide.

EDEMA is swelling in any part or all of the body due to the abnormal accumulation of excess fluid.

EDIBLE PORTION (EP) is the part of a food normally eaten, in contrast to the waste portion such as bones, gristle, peels, stems and seeds.

EDTA (ethylenediaminetetraacetic acid) is a nonspecific chelating agent or substance that binds with minerals like calcium, copper, iron or zinc and keeps them from reacting with other substances. It is used as a food additive to stabilize and keep fats, oil, shellfish, meats and dairy products fresh. Medically, EDTA is used to treat lead poisoning. It has been used in questionable therapy for atherosclerosis.

See Chelation, Processing agents

EGG SUBSTITUTES, containing mainly egg whites, are often recommended for low cholesterol diets as they contain no cholesterol. An egg yolk contains about 250 mg of cholesterol. A typical egg substitute is ninety-nine percent egg white along with corn oil, vegetable gums, artificial colors, emulsifiers, minerals and vitamins. The vitamin and mineral content of the egg substitute and the egg are similar. In many recipes, two egg whites can be substituted for one whole egg, eliminating the egg yolk and its cholesterol content.

Egg substitute	Whole egg
¼ cup (55 gm)	1 egg (44 gm)
25 Calories	70 Calories
5 gm protein	5 gm protein
1 gm carbohydrate	1 gm carbohydrate
0 gm fat	5 gm fat
0 mg cholesterol	240 mg cholesterol
80 mg sodium	60 mg sodium

ELIMINATION DIETS are used to diagnose food sensitivity. For one week a very limited selection of foods is given. For example, rice and lamb are often first eaten because they are least likely to cause reactions. By the fifth or sixth day of the elimination diet, allergic symptoms will be gone if the person is truly sensitive to some food. Then single food challenges are introduced, one at a time, for two days at a time to identify the offending foods.

See Allergy

-EMIA, or *aemia,* is a suffix relating to a condition of the blood or presence in the blood of a substance.

EMPTY CALORIE FOODS usually refer to foods that supply calories from sugar or fat but contain little or no other nutrients. Some candies, chips and pastries fall into this category. Eating small amounts of these foods is all right for most of us, but excess use can crowd out more nutritious choices.

ENRICHED refers to the process by which flour nutrients lost during refinement are added back to refined breads and cereals. Thiamin (B_1), niacin and iron are added back at levels about equal to those in the whole grain. Riboflavin (B_2) is added back at levels about twice that found in the original whole grain. These levels are regulated by federal law and monitored by the FDA, so that when a bread or cereal claims to be enriched the consumer is assured of what and how much of each nutrient has been added to the food. Enrichment does not restore all the nutrients found in the whole grain. This term is often used synonymously with "fortified" but technically they do not mean the same thing.

See Fortified

ENZYMES are substances produced in living cells that speed up metabolic reactions without being used up in the process. We produce thousands of different enzymes. The names of many begin with the name of the substance they act on and end in "ase." An example is lactase, an enzyme that digests milk sugar lactose.

Most enzymes are made up of protein (apoenzyme) and a nonprotein portion, usually a vitamin or mineral.

EPA (eicosapentanoic acid) and DHA (docosahex-

anoic acid) (sometimes called fish oils) are polyunsaturated fatty acids found in high levels in fish. Research has shown that people who eat fish have a lower incidence of coronary heart disease. The fish oils reduce levels of fat in the blood, reduce clotting and may decrease formation of plaque in the arteries. Experts suggest that eating fish only once or twice a week could help prevent coronary heart disease. These fatty acids have also been found to be antiinflammatory so they may prove useful for disorders like arthritis.

Salmon, mackeral, anchovies, cod and cod liver oil are good sources of EPA and DHA. Fish oil is also sold as a supplement in capsules.

EQUAL, *see* Aspartame

ESSENTIAL FATTY ACID, *see* Linoleic acid

EVENING PRIMROSE OIL (rampion) is a plant oil rich in linoleic acid. Linoleic acid is a polyunsaturated fatty acid that must be obtained in the diet as it cannot be made in the body. It is sometimes recommended for eczema and lowering cholesterol but its value for either of these uses has not yet been established.

See Polyunsaturated fat

F

FAST FOODS are ready-to-eat food items available with little or no waiting time. Names like Wendy's, Roy Rogers, Pizza Hut, Taco Bell and Burger King come to mind instantly. Seven percent of the U.S. population eats in a McDonald's daily. Currently there are over 140,000 fast food restaurants, independently owned or managed by the more than 340 national and regional fast food restaurant chains.

The major drawback to fast foods is that many choices are very high in calories, fat, salt and sugar, and low in fiber and some vitamins and minerals. With more careful selections—milk instead of a soft drink, a plain hamburger instead of one with all the trimmings, or a salad with a little dressing rather than French fries—a fast food meal can be a useful contribution to your day's food intake.

The following analysis of fast foods gives a calorie and nutrient breakdown of some representative menu items from popular food chains.

Summary of Selected Fast Food Nutrient Data

HAMBURGERS

Burger King

	Calories	Protein (grams)	Fat (grams)	Carbohydrates (grams)	Sodium (mg)	Cholesterol (mg)	Percentage U.S. RDA[a] Protein	Vitamin A	Vitamin C	Calcium	Iron
Hamburger	310	16	12	35	560	NA	25	2	2	6	15
Cheeseburger	360	18	16	35	705	NA	30	6	2	15	15
Whopper	670	27	38	56	975	NA	40	10	20	10	25
Whopper w/cheese	760	33	45	56	1260	NA	50	20	20	25	30
Bacon Double Cheeseburger	600	35	35	36	985	NA	50	8	2	25	25
Whopper Jr.	370	16	18	35	545	NA	25	6	8	6	15
Whopper Jr. w/cheese	410	19	21	35	685	NA	30	8	8	15	15

(Burger King Corporation suggests that to reduce calorie levels of a Whopper by about 153 or a Whopper Jr. by about 51, order the sandwich without mayonnaise. To reduce the sodium level of a hamburger or cheeseburger by about 93 mg, a Whopper by about 186 mg, or a Whopper Jr. by about 93 mg, order the sandwich without pickles.)

81

HAMBURGERS

	Calories	Protein (grams)	Fat (grams)	Carbohydrates (grams)	Sodium (mg)	Cholesterol (mg)	Percentage U.S. RDA[a]				
							Protein	Vitamin A	Vitamin C	Calcium	Iron
Jack in the Box											
Hamburger	263	13	11	29	565	26	30	*	2	8	15
Cheeseburger	310	16	15	28	875	32	35	6	*	15	15
Jumbo Jack Hamburger	551	28	20	45	1135	80	60	4	6	15	25
Arby's											
Regular Roast Beef	350	22	15	32	880	45	35	*	*	8	20
Super Roast Beef	620	30	28	61	1420	85	45	*	*	10	30
Beef 'N Cheddar	484	29	21	46	1745	70	45	4	*	25	10
Jack in the Box											
Regular Taco	190	8	11	15	460	20	20	6	*	10	6
Super Taco	280	12	17	20	970	35	25	10	2	20	10
Roy Rogers											
Roast Beef Sandwich	317	27	10	29	785	55	60	2	*	9	23
Roast Beef Sandwich w/cheese	424	33	19	30	1694	77	73	8	*	34	24
Large Roast Beef	360	34	12	30	1044	73	75	2	*	9	26
Large Roast Beef w/cheese	467	40	21	30	1953	95	88	8	*	34	27

Taco Bell

Beef Burrito	466	30	21	37	327	NA	45	34	25	8	26
Burrito Supreme	457	21	22	43	367	NA	30	69	27	12	21
Tostada	179	9	6	25	101	NA	15	63	16	19	13
Taco	186	15	8	14	79	NA	25	2	*	12	14

Wendy's

Chili	260	21	8	26	1070	30	30	20	10	8	25
Taco Salad	390	23	18	36	1100	40	35	35	35	20	25

CHICKEN

Arby's

Chicken Breast Sandwich	584	27	28	55	1323	56	40	*	*	10	20

Burger King

Chicken Sandwich	690	26	42	52	775	NA	40	4	2	6	10

Church's Fried Chicken

Breast	278	21	17	9	560	NA	47	NA	NA	NA	NA
Wing	178	22	20	9	583	NA	48	NA	NA	NA	NA
Thigh	306	18	22	9	448	NA	41	NA	NA	NA	NA
Leg	147	13	9	4	286	NA	28	NA	NA	NA	NA

Kentucky Fried Chicken

Original Recipe (2 pieces)	393	28	26	11	868	164	60	*	*	6	12
Original Recipe Dinner	661	33	38	48	1536	172	75	5	61	13	21

	Calories	Protein (grams)	Fat (grams)	Carbohydrates (grams)	Sodium (mg)	Cholesterol (mg)	protein (mg)	Vitamin A	Vitamin C	Calcium	Iron
								Percentage U.S. RDA[a]			
CHICKEN											
Extra Crispy (2 pieces)	544	32	37	21	861	168	70	*	*	6	12
Extra Crispy Dinner	902	36	48	58	1529	176	80	5	61	14	36
(Dinners include 2 pieces chicken, mashed potatoes, gravy, cole slaw and roll. Nutritional values for fried chicken vary for different chicken parts and for pieces of different sizes. These figures are based on a typical combination of 1 wing and 1 thigh.)											
McDonald's											
Chicken McNuggets (6 pieces, without sauce)	314	20	19	15	525	76	45	*	*	1	6
Wendy's											
Chicken Sandwich (on multi-grain bun)	320	25	10	31	500	59	35	*	*	2	8
FISH											
Arthur Treacher's											
Fish (2 pieces)	360	19	20	25	450	56	30	*	2	2	2

84

Shrimp (7 pieces)	380	13	21	27	538	93	20	*	2	6	4
Chowder	110	5	3	11	835	9	7	6	2	6	*
Fish Sandwich	444	16	15	40	836	42	25	*	2	8	2
Burger King											
Whaler	540	24	24	57	745	NA	35	*	*	8	15
Whaler w/cheese	590	26	28	58	885	NA	40	4	*	20	15
Long John Silver's											
Fish w/batter (1 piece)	202	13	12	11	673	31	28	NA	NA	NA	NA
Baked fish w/sauce	151	33	2	0	361	90	73	NA	NA	NA	NA
Catfish fillet	203	12	12	13	469	49	27	NA	NA	NA	NA
Breaded clams	526	17	31	58	1170	2	37	NA	NA	NA	NA
Fish Sandwich	555	20	33	45	1242	48	44	NA	NA	NA	NA
McDonald's											
Filet-O-Fish	432	14	25	37	781	47	30	4	*	9	10
OTHER ENTREES											
Arby's											
Ham 'N Cheese	484	29	21	46	1745	70	45	4	*	25	10
Arthur Treacher's											
Krunch Pup	203	5	26	12	446	25	8	*	6	*	2

	Calories	Protein (grams)	Fat (grams)	Carbohydrates (grams)	Sodium (mg)	Cholesterol (mg)	Percentage U.S. RDA[a]				
							Protein	Vitamin A	Vitamin C	Calcium	Iron
OTHER ENTREES											
Burger King											
Ham and Cheese Sandwich	550	29	30	43	1550	NA	45	20	25	25	25
Veal Parmagiana	580	36	27	46	805	NA	45	20	30	25	25
Dairy Queen/Brazier											
Hot Dog	280	11	16	21	830	45	15	*	*	8	8
Hot Dog w/Chili	320	13	20	23	985	55	20	*	*	8	10
Hot Dog w/Cheese	330	15	21	21	990	55	20	2	*	15	8
Super Hot Dog	520	17	27	44	1365	80	25	*	*	15	15
Pizza Hut											
Standard Cheese Pizza (½ 13" medium, Thin 'N Crispy)	680	38	22	84	1800	NA	80	24	*	100	40
Supreme Pizza (½ 13" medium, Thin 'N Crispy)	800	42	34	88	2400	NA	90	30	8	80	50
Taco Bell											
Bean Burrito	343	11	12	48	272	NA	15	33	25	10	16

POTATOES

Burger King											
French fries	210	3	11	25	230	NA	4	*	4	*	2
Kentucky Fried Chicken											
Mashed potatoes w/gravy	87	2	3	14	325	1	3	*	8	2	3
McDonald's											
Regular fries	220	3	12	26	109	9	5	*	21	*	3
Roy Rogers											
Baked potatoes											
Plain	211	6	+	48	65	0	13	*	45	2	9
w/oleo	274	6	7	48	161	0	13	6	56	2	9
w/sour cream 'n chives	408	7	21	48	138	31	11	10	26	10	13
w/broccoli 'n cheese	376	14	18	40	523	19	21	4	14	21	14
w/taco beef 'n cheese	463	22	22	45	726	37	33	5	22	15	21
Wendy's											
French fries	280	4	14	35	95	15	6	NA	20	*	6
Baked potatoes											
Plain	250	6	2	52	60	0	8	*	60	2	15
w/sour cream & chives	460	6	24	53	230	15	8	10	60	4	15
w/cheese	590	17	34	55	450	22	35	20	60	35	15

	Calories	Protein (grams)	Fat (grams)	Carbohydrates (grams)	Sodium (mg)	Cholesterol (mg)	Percentage U.S. RDA[a]				
							Protein	Vitamin A	Vitamin C	Calcium	Iron
POTATOES											
w/chili & cheese	510	22	20	63	610	22	40	15	60	25	20
w/bacon & cheese	570	19	30	57	1180	22	35	15	60	20	15
w/broccoli & cheese	500	13	25	54	430	22	20	35	150	25	15
OTHER SIDE DISHES											
Burger King											
Onion rings	270	3	16	29	450	NA	4	*	*	2	2
Kentucky Fried Chicken											
Cole slaw	121	1	8	13	225	7	*	5	53	3	3
Long John Silver's											
Corn on the cob	176	5	4	29	0	0	8	NA	NA	NA	NA
Hush puppies (2)	145	3	7	18	405	1	5	NA	NA	NA	NA
DESSERTS											
Burger King											
Apple pie	330	3	14	48	385	NA	4	*	2	*	2

Item											
Long John Silver's											
Pecan pie	446	5	22	59	435	92	10	NA	NA	NA	NA
Roy Rogers											
Hot fudge sundae	337	6	12	53	186	23	14	10	*	26	5
SHAKES											
Burger King											
Vanilla	340	8	11	52	320	NA	10	*	*	30	*
Jack in the Box											
Strawberry	380	11	10	63	268	33	25	8	*	35	2
McDonald's											
Chocolate	383	10	9	66	300	30	20	7	*	32	5
Wendy's											
Frosty (12 oz.)	400	8	14	59	220	50	20	10	*	30	6
OTHER BEVERAGES											
Cola (12 oz.)	145	0	0	37	NA	0	*	*	*	*	*
Diet soft drink (12 oz.)	1	0	0	0	NA	0	*	*	*	*	*
Milk (whole, 8 oz.)	150	8	8	11	120	33	20	6	4	30	*
Coffee (black)	0	0	0	0	NA	0	*	*	*	*	*
BREAKFAST ITEMS											
McDonald's											
Egg McMuffin	327	18	15	31	885	229	40	12	*	23	16

	Calories	Protein (grams)	Fat (grams)	Carbohydrates (grams)	Sodium (mg)	Cholesterol (mg)	Percentage U.S. RDA [a]				
							Protein	Vitamin A	Vitamin C	Calcium	Iron
BREAKFAST ITEMS											
Scrambled Egg Breakfast (includes scrambled eggs, sausage, English muffin w/butter, and hash brown potatoes)	697	28	44	47	1463	412	60	16	10	20	29
Hotcakes and Sausage (w/butter and syrup)	706	17	29	94	1685	90	25	5	8	12	17
English muffin (w/butter)	186	5	5	30	318	13	8	3	*	12	8
Hash brown potatoes	125	2	7	14	325	7	3	*	7	*	2
Orange Juice (6 oz.)	80	1	0	20	0	0	*	8	140	*	*
Roy Rogers											
Crescent sandwich	401	13	27	25	867	148	30	10	*	16	9
w/bacon	431	15	30	26	1035	156	34	10	*	16	9
w/sausage	449	20	30	26	1289	168	44	10	*	16	10
w/ham	557	20	42	25	1192	189	44	10	*	17	12

Apple Danish	249	4	12	32	255	15	7	2	*	10	7
Cheese Danish	254	5	12	31	260	11	8	2	*	4	6
Wendy's											
Breakfast Sandwich	370	17	19	33	770	200	30	15	NA	15	20
French Toast	400	11	19	45	850	115	15	10	NA	8	10
Home Fries	360	4	22	37	745	20	6	NA	8	2	4

NA—Data not available.
*less than 2 percent
+less than 1 gram

[a] The U.S. RDA (U.S. Recommended Daily Allowance) is the standard used for nutrition labeling and is meant to apply to almost all Americans 4 years of age and older. It is derived from the RDA (Recommended Dietary Allowances) described in the text of this report by using the RDA for the sex-age group which has the *highest* nutrient requirement. For most nutrients, this group is teenage boys. (Pregnant and lactating women are not included. They, infants, and children under the age of 4 are covered by separate U.S. RDAs.)

[b] The U.S. RDA for high quality protein (such as that found in eggs and other animal products) is 45 grams, and for lower quality protein (found in vegetable sources) is 65 grams.

[c] The data on Taco Bell items were calculated, rather than derived from analysis. Taco Bell cannot guarantee their accuracy.

[d] Information derived from U.S. Department of Agriculture data.

COURTESY: American Council on Science and Health, from *Fast Food and the American Diet*, 1985.

FASTING, or going without food, is used for losing weight and for spiritual and physical purposes, for religious reasons and as a form of protest. Everyone, or at least most of us, fast between meals and during the night. Short-term fasting for a day or so is safe for healthy people. Fasting for longer periods should be medically supervised.

During the early stages of fasting, liver glycogen is broken down to supply glucose for energy. Fat is released from body stores along with protein from muscle, which is converted into energy. Ketone bodies formed from the breakdown of body fats can be used for energy by most body tissues after an adaptation period of about three days. If fasting continues, the body's metabolic rate decreases so that less energy is needed, slowing down weight loss. Extreme obesity has been successfully treated with medically supervised fasting conducted in a hospital.

See Ketosis

FAT is a more concentrated source of calories than carbohydrate or protein, yielding 9 Calories per gram. Besides energy, fat also provides essential fatty acids (which the body cannot make), insulates the body, protects vital organs, carries fat soluble vitamins, is part of cell membranes, and makes food taste good. Approximately 98 percent of fat in foods and 90 percent of fat in the body are triglycerides. There are many different triglycerides but they are all made up of glycerol and three fatty acids. The kind of fatty acids determines the type of fat. Fatty acids are chains of two to twenty carbon atoms. Their length and degree of saturation help to determine the physical characteristics of the fat. When the chain has less than six carbons it is a short chain fatty acid. Medium chain fatty acids contain eight to ten carbon atoms and long chain fatty acids have twelve carbons or more. The

Chemical Structure of Fats

(A) **Saturated** (stearic acid)

(B) **Monounsaturated** (oleic acid)

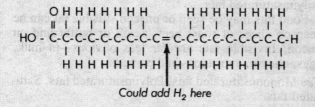

Could add H₂ here

(C) **Polyunsaturated** (linoleic acid)

Could add H₂ here

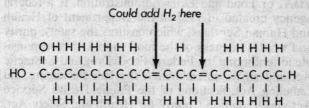

longer the chain, the higher the temperature needed to melt the fat.

The fatty acids can be saturated, monounsaturated or polyunsaturated. This refers to the ratio of hydrogen atoms to carbon atoms. When the fatty acid is holding all the hydrogen atoms it can it is said to be saturated (see A, p. 93). These are mostly animal fats. When there is room to add on more hydrogen atoms, that fatty acid is unsaturated. Monounsaturated fatty acids can have two more hydrogen atoms (note the double bond in the structure), while polyunsaturated fatty acids can have many more additional hydrogen atoms added (see B and C, p. 93).

Vegetable fats contain mainly monounsaturated and polyunsaturated fats.

Food fats may be seen or unseen. Visible fat can be seen on slices of roast beef, as oil or butter and on bacon. Invisible fats are far less obvious—in milk, eggs, cheese, avocadoes and peanuts.

See Monounsaturated fats, Polyunsaturated fats, Saturated fats

FATTY ACIDS, *see* Fats

FDA, or Food and Drug Administration, is a federal agency created in 1927 in the Department of Health and Human Services, which ensures the safety, purity and wholesomeness of the food supply. It is responsible for enforcing the Federal Food, Drug and Cosmetic Act and all its amendments, the Fair Packaging and Labeling Act, sections of the Public Health Service Act and Radiation Control for Health and Safety Act. It protects Americans from injury, unsanitary food and fraud by analyzing samples, conducting inspections, and doing research on toxicity, chemical contamination, pesticide residues and long-term drug effects. The FDA approves new food additives before they are used and reviews additives currently in use. It controls communicable disease by controlling the movement of food across state lines. Nutrition labeling is also under the direction of the FDA. It also supports the individual states' programs for shellfish and milk safety.

See Nutrition labeling

FD&C APPROVED FOOD COLORS refers to synthetic color additives that have been approved for use in food. The abbreviation FD&C stands for food, drug and cosmetic, indicating intended use for the coloring agents. Colors are added to foods to make them more appealing. Colors are added to soft drinks, ice creams, sherbets, gelatin, puddings, cake mixes, baked goods, candy and even pet foods. Some colors are natural, coming from foods—for example, carotenes, caramel, chlorophyll, annatto seeds, tumeric, beets. However, most of the food colors—about 90 percent of all that are used—are synthetic.

At the present time, there are nine certified colors and two of these have limited use. Citrus Red No. 2 is limited to use in orange skins and FD&C Red No. 4 is limited to maraschino cherries. FD&C Blue No. 1, FD&C Blue No. 2, FD&C Green No. 3, FD&C Red No. 3, FD&C Red No. 40, FD&C Yellow No. 5 and FD&C Yellow No. 6 are the seven colors currently approved with no limitations. When FD&C Yellow No. 5 (tartrazine) is used in a product, it must be identified on the label and not listed simply as an artificial color. This is required because some people have experienced severe allergic reactions to this color and need to avoid foods containing it. Persons who are affected by aspirin may be sensitive to Yellow No. 5.

See Artificial colors, Natural food colors

FEINGOLD DIET is a diet that eliminates synthetic food colors and flavors, preservatives and salicylates (aspirinlike substances). It is used to treat hyperactivity in children. Hyperactive children have short attention spans, cannot concentrate and are disruptive in school and at home. A pediatric allergist, Dr. Benjamin Feingold, believed that hyperactivity (also called hyperkinesis or ADD, attention deficit disorder) was due to a reaction to these substances. He claimed that 50 percent of his patients were helped by a diet restricted in these compounds. The diet was difficult to follow as most foods contain some amount of salicylates and many foods contain artificial colors, flavors and preservatives. After a while Dr. Feingold singled out artificial colors as the main offenders. This restriction alone would cut out luncheon meats, most ice creams, pudding, candies and even nonfood items like toothpaste and some vitamin pills. Eating in restaurants and school cafeterias is almost impossible. The value of this restrictive diet has been tested and on the basis of many carefully controlled studies, the diet appears to be effective in only a very small percentage of children, usually preschoolers. In some genetically predisposed children, hyperactivity can be caused by Red dye No. 3.

FETAL ALCOHOL SYNDROME refers to physical and mental defects seen in infants whose mothers drank alcohol during pregnancy. The defects include low birth weight, heart problems, poor growth, mental retardation, facial deformities (particularly in eyelids and upper lip) and hyperactivity. The exact amount of alcohol that could cause problems has not yet been determined. The stage (trimester) of pregnancy when the alcohol is consumed is also a factor. Alcohol use in the first trimester may cause miscarriage and abnormal organ formation. During the second trimester skeletal growth is affected. Drinking near the end of pregnancy causes low birth weight babies. Because of this uncertainty, the American College of Obstetricians and Gynecologists recommends that no alcohol be drunk during pregnancy.

FEVER refers to an elevation of body temperature above 98.6°F (37°C). Fever is the body's response to toxins produced by an infection or inflammation. The fever causes an increase in the calories needed, as metabolic rate increases seven percent for each degree Fahrenheit rise (thirteen percent for each degree Celsius rise). The heat production uses up more calories and added to this are extra calories used because a feverish person is often restless. The fever also causes an increased loss of body water due to sweating; as many as ten cups of liquid a day may be needed to compensate for the loss. Some experts recommend a small vitamin C supplement during a fever as stress increases the body's use of this vitamin.

The old saying "starve a fever" is far from correct. If the feverish person doesn't feel like eating, he should be given liquids that contain calories—for example, fruit juice, lemonade, or sweetened tea.

FEVER BLISTERS, or herpes simplex, of the lips, are sometimes called cold sores because they often occur when a person has a cold, lacks sleep or is in a rundown condition. Lysine, an essential amino acid, has been effective in treating cold sores. A combination of bioflavinoids and vitamin C (200 mg of each taken three times a day) has been effective when used just as the blisters are starting to form. In many cases the fever blisters will not erupt, or if they do, they will last a much shorter time than usual.

FIBER is a type of carbohydrate that cannot be digested. It is found in plant foods like whole grains, fruit and vegetables. Fibrous material in meat is protein and can be digested. Good sources of fiber are whole wheat bread, unprocessed bran, grapes, popcorn, beans and carrots. Regular intake of adequate fiber is useful in maintaining normal bowel movements. Other benefits claimed for high fiber intake—lowered incidence of

Dietary Fiber in Foods

Food	Portion	Grams of dietary fiber*
Apple, unpeeled	1 medium	5.67
Apple, peeled	1 medium	1.96
Banana	1 small	2.08
Baked beans	½ cup	9.27
Bran	1 tablespoon	1.80
Bread, white	1 slice	.68
Bread, whole-wheat	1 slice	2.13
Broccoli, cooked	½ cup	3.18
Cabbage, cooked	½ cup	2.50
Cauliflower, cooked	½ cup	.42
Carrots, cooked	½ cup	2.87
Cereals		
All-Bran	1 ounce	4.00
Corn Flakes	½ cup	1.38
Grape-Nuts	¼ cup	2.10
Shredded Wheat	1 biscuit	3.07
Special K	½ cup	.82
Sugar Puffs	½ cup	.91
Corn, canned	½ cup	4.69
Lettuce	⅙ head	1.53
Peanut butter	1 tablespoon	1.21
Peach, fresh, unpeeled	1	2.28
Pear, unpeeled	1	12.59
Peas, cooked	½ cup	6.67
Strawberries	1 cup	2.65
Tomatoes	1 medium	1.89

*Recommended intakes of dietary fiber are between 30 and 40 grams daily.

colon and other cancer, diverticulosis, appendicitis and others—have yet to be proven. In spite of this it would probably be a good idea, however, for most of us to increase our intake of fiber.

PUT A LITTLE FIBER (BULK) IN YOUR LIFE

Step 1: Eat whole-grain breads and cereals.
For the first few days eat one serving of whole-grain breads, cereal, pasta or brown rice. Gradually increase to four or more servings daily.

Step 2: Eat fresh fruits and vegetables.
Begin by eating one serving a day of a raw, unpeeled fruit or cooked vegetables including skins. Gradually increase to four servings a day.

Step 3: Eat dried peas and beans.
Begin by eating one serving a week (split pea soup, lentils, baked beans, peanuts) and let your taste be your guide. We'd suggest at least two to three servings a week.

Step 4: Eat unprocessed bran.
Add bran to your food—cereal, soup, casseroles, muffins, pancakes, baked goods. Start with one teaspoon a day and over a three-week period gradually work up to two to three tablespoons daily. Remember, large amounts of bran are not needed; and drink plenty of liquids along with bran.

FIBROCYSTIC BREAST DISEASE describes the presence of lumps or fluid-filled cysts in the breast. These can be quite painful, especially before and during the menstrual period. All breast lumps should be evaluated by a physician. Eliminating caffeine in coffee, soft drinks and other foods and medicines and taking 600 IU of vitamin E daily for eight weeks, have been suggested to reduce the lumps.

See Caffeine

FISH is a nutritious food, rich in good quality protein, and low in fat. Even fatty fish like salmon and mackeral contain less fat than red meat. Shellfish are very low in fat. Fish are also sources of many vitamins and minerals—especially niacin (a B vitamin) as one serving supplies 50 percent of the daily requirement.

Calories in Fish*

Finfish	Calories in 3½ ounces (cooked)
Bass, striped, broiled	228
Bluefish, filet, baked	160
Cod, broiled	162
Croaker, baked	133
Eel	233
Fishsticks, frozen†	176
Flounder, baked	202
Haddock, broiled	141
Herring, kippered	211
Mackerel, broiled	300
Pompano, broiled	284
Roe, baked	126
Salmon, canned	203
Sardines, canned in oil	311
Trout, cooked	196
Tuna, canned in oil	288
Tuna, canned in water	127
Shellfish	
Clams, raw	82
Crab, steamed	93
Lobster, canned	88
Oysters, raw	66
Scallops, steamed	112
Shrimp, canned	80

*Cooked without added fat or coating.
†Commercially prepared with coating.

Americans do not eat very much fish. On the average we eat less than 15 pounds each in a year, compared with the consumption of 66 pounds of poultry and over 150 pounds of meat per person.

Fish are recommended in low-fat, low-cholesterol diets. The cholesterol content of shellfish is not an issue as it is now estimated to be lower than it had been believed to be. Earlier estimates included total sterols (fatty substances) in the shellfish, and only 35 to 45 percent of these are cholesterol.

Fish eating has been found beneficial in reducing the risk of cardiovascular disease. Fish eating populations have less incidence of heart disease.

Below is a chart showing the calorie content of commonly eaten fish.

See EPA

FISH OILS, *see* EPA

FLATULENCE, *see* Gas

FLAVORING AGENTS make up the largest single class of food additives which includes natural and synthetic flavors, spices, essential oils, flavor enhancers and sweeteners. Sugar, salt and corn syrup are the three most used food additives accounting for 130 of the 140 pounds of additives consumed per person yearly. Following is a list of commonly used flavoring agents.

Additive	Used in	Function
Artificial flavoring	soda pop	flavoring
	candy	
	breakfast cereal	
	gelatin desserts	
	many processed	
	foods	

Additive	Used in	Function
Aspartame	cold breakfast cereal	noncaloric sweetener
	chewing gum	
	drink mixes	
	instant coffee and tea	
	gelatin	
	pudding	
	pie filling	
	nondairy whipped topping	
Corn syrup corn syrup solids	candy	sweetener
	toppings	thickener
	syrup	
	snack food	
	imitation dairy foods	
	coffee whitener	
Dextrose glucose corn sugar	bread	sweetener
	caramel	coloring agent
	soft drinks	
	cookies	
	many processed foods	
Fumaric acid	powdered drinks	tartness agent
	pudding	
	pie filling	
	gelatin desserts	
Hydrolyzed vegetable protein (HVP)	instant soups	flavor enhancer
	frankfurters	
	sauce mixes	
	beef stew	

Additive	Used in	Function
Invert sugar	candy soft drinks many processed foods	sweetener
Lactose	whipped topping mix breakfast pastry	sweetener
Mannitol	chewing gum low-calorie food	sweetener
Monosodium glutamate (MSG)	soup seafood poultry cheese sauces many processed foods	flavor enhancer
Quinine	tonic water quinine water bitter lemon	flavoring
Saccharin	diet food and drinks	noncaloric sweetener
Salt sodium chloride	most processed food	flavoring
Sorbitol	diet food and drinks candy shredded coconut chewing gum	sweetener thickening agent maintains moisture
Sugar sucrose	table sugar sweetened food	sweetener

Additive	Used in	Function

Vanillin
    ethyl vanillin
	ice cream
	baked goods
	beverages
	chocolate
	candy
	gelatin desserts
		substitute for va-
		    nilla

FLAVORINGS are substances that stimulate our sense of taste and smell. We can taste four main flavors—sweet, salty, bitter and sour—via the taste buds on our tongues. We have approximately 10,000 of these taste receptors. The variety of flavors we enjoy results from combinations of these four tastes and the varying odors of foods.

Most natural flavorings are made from plants. Synthetic flavorings can be made that are very similar to these. In fact, persons allergic to strawberries sometimes react to artificial strawberry flavoring too!

Sugar and salt make up 140 to 150 pounds of the additives eaten annually per person in the United States. Both are natural flavorings. Other flavoring agents are eaten in smaller amounts.

FLUORIDATION refers to the addition of trace amounts (0.5 to 1.0 part per million) of fluoride, usually as sodium fluoride, to drinking water, to protect against dental caries (cavities). More than 100 million Americans live in communities where the public water supply has been fluoridated, resulting in a 60 percent or more reduction in tooth decay. Not only does fluoride protect teeth, but it makes the bones of older adults more resistent to osteoporosis (adult bone loss).

Opponents of fluoridation claim that when this mineral is put in the water supply there are higher incidences of cancer, cardiovascular disease and Down's syndrome. None of these claims have held up under careful scientific investigation.

See Dental disease, Fluoride, Osteoporosis

FLUORIDE is a mineral widely, but unevenly, found in many foods. Seafood and tea are the richest sources. Fluoride is an essential nutrient needed for sound bones and teeth. The Recommended Dietary Allowance suggests that a safe and adequate daily intake is 1.5 to 4.0 mg. In areas where the water supply is fluoridated this amount is easy to obtain. The daily intake in many parts of the United States is not sufficient to protect against tooth decay. In those areas infants and children should be given fluoride supplementation.

Too much fluoride can be dangerous. When a person takes in 20 mg a day or more for an extended period of time, fluorosis will occur. This is fluoride poisoning which results in mottled, irregularly worn teeth with eventual softening and deformity of the bones and teeth. Poisoning can also result from a large, single dose of fluoride. This is unlikely in adults but young children have been known to eat or drink brightly colored, minty, fluoride-containing toothpastes and mouthwashes. Generally these items are left within easy reach since they are not considered hazardous. Many mouthwashes, high in fluoride, have a warning on the label not to swallow or to be used by children under the age of six.

See Fluoridation, Minerals.

FOLIC ACID (folacin, folate) is part of the B complex family of vitamins. It is part of a coenzyme that acts in many metabolic reactions in the body. Folic acid deficiency causes a type of anemia in which the red blood cells are larger than normal. Pregnant women are

Sources of Folic Acid

Food	Amount	Milligrams
Product 19, Kellogg's	1 cup	.40
Brewer's yeast	1 tablespoon	.31
Orange juice	1 cup	.16
Romaine lettuce, chopped	1 cup	.10
Brussels sprouts	3 large	.10
Carnation Breakfast Bar	1	.10
Crispix, Kellogg's	¾ cup	.10
Cocoa Krispies, Kellogg's	1 cup	.10
Beets	2 medium	.09
Sweet potato	1 medium	.08
Asparagus	5–6 spears	.06
Orange	1 medium	.06
Wheat germ	¼ cup	.05
Cantaloupe, diced	1 cup	.05
Grapefruit juice	½ cup	.05
Milk, regular	1 cup	.04
Red pepper	1 medium	.04
Avocado	½ medium	.04
Yogurt	8 ounces	.03
Beer	12 ounces	.03
Cucumber	1 small	.03
Cabbage	½ cup	.02
Potato	1 medium	.02
Strawberries	1 cup	.02
Whole-wheat bread	1 slice	.02

The RDA for folic acid is: 0.4 mg

The U.S. RDA (labeling tool) for folic acid is: 0.4 mg

particularly vulnerable to this condition because of their increased need for the vitamin. Other symptoms of deficiency can be sore tongue, fainting, diarrhea and weight loss.

The RDA is 400 mcg for adults; that requirement is doubled in pregnancy. Only 200 to 250 mcg of folic acid are contained in the usual American diet: Green leafy vegetables like spinach, beet greens and asparagus, liver, wheat germ and orange juice are good sources.

Sickle cell anemia, leukemia and psoriasis are often treated with medications that antagonize folic acid. Vitamin supplements should not be taken in these situations without a physician's approval.

The amount of folic acid in nonprescription vitamin supplements is regulated. No more than 400 mcg (800 mcg in prenatal supplements) is allowed. This is to prevent the possibility that excess folic acid could cover up a more serious form of anemia.

See Anemia, Vitamins

FOOD is anything one thinks is edible. Edible items are determined by the cultural group one belongs to. In northern China women and first-born sons are not permitted to eat eggs; Bantu women of child-bearing age are forbidden to drink milk as it is believed to cause infertility. Roast dog meat is an acceptable choice in many areas in the world, yet, here in the United States, when an army officer killed and roasted a dog to demonstrate military survival, he was prosecuted and fined $200 for cruelty to animals.

What people are allowed to eat, when, where and in what combinations, are one's food habits—an integral part of all cultures. A culture's food habits help to standardize behavior to promote the homogenieity of a designated group of people. Food habits are learned and continue to change as a reflection of the needs of the group taking into account the availability of food, religious beliefs and practices, sanitation and social customs.

FOOD ALLERGY is an unusual or exaggerated response to a food. It can occur immediately or be delayed for as long as five days after eating. Signs of food allergy range from nausea, vomiting, diarrhea, sneezing, itching, eczema, canker sores, headache, rash, hives to total body shock, a very rare reaction. Some allergists believe that behavioral problems like hyperactivity, tension and fatigue are caused by food allergies.

Any food can cause an allergic reaction in a sensitive person. Milk, eggs, wheat, peanuts, soybeans, nuts, fish, shellfish and chocolate are common offenders. If a person is sensitive to one member of a food family he may also react to other members.

See Elimination diet

Common Food Allergen Families

Food groups	Possible reactions
Milk (whole, dried, skim, buttermilk, cheese, custard, cream, creamed foods, yogurt, ice cream, sherbet, ice milk, goat's milk)	Indigestion, constipation, diarrhea, gas, abdominal pain, nasal congestion, bronchial congestion, sore throat, ear inflammation, asthma, headache, bad breath, sweating, tension, fatigue
Kola nut (chocolate, cola beverage)	Headache, asthma, indigestion, chronic nasal inflammation, skin inflammation, itching

Food groups	Possible reactions
Corn (corn, corn syrup, corn cereal, popcorn, Cracker Jacks, grits, corn chips, cornstarch, cornmeal, corn oil[a])	Irritability, insomnia, oversensitivity, restlessness, allergic fatigue,[b] headache
Egg (eggs, French toast, baked goods, icing, meringue, candies, creamy salad dressing, breaded food, noodles, egg substitutes, egg odor)	Hives, eczema, asthma, indigestion, headache
Pea family—legumes[c] (peanuts, peanut butter, dried peas, dried beans, honey,[d] licorice, soybean, soy flour, soy protein, soy milk, soy oil,[a] alfalfa)	Asthma, hives, headache
Citrus fruits[e] (orange, lemon, lime, grapefruit, tangerine)	Eczema, hives, asthma, canker sores
Tomato (ketchup, chili, prepared foods)	Eczema, hives, asthma, mouth soreness
Wheat and small grains[c] (rice, barley, oats, wild rice, millet, rye[a])	Asthma, indigestion, eczema, nasal congestion, bronchial congestion
Cinnamon[f] (ketchup, chewing gum, candies, baked goods, applesauce, apple pies	Hives, headache, asthma

Food groups	Possible reactions
and cakes, chili, luncheon meats, pumpkin pies and cakes)	
Artificial food colors (yellow dye tartrazine, FD&C #5, colored foods, colored drinks, colored medicines)	Asthma, hives

[a] Only an occasional offender.
[b] Characterized by unresponsiveness, sleepiness, vague aching, weakness.
[c] Reactions to this group are severe, including shock.
[d] In the United States, honey is gathered primarily from plants in this family (i.e., clover, alfalfa).
[e] If the person is sensitive to citric acid, he or she will also react to tart artificial drinks and pineapple.
[f] Cinnamon-sensitive patients cannot tolerate bay leaf.

FOOD GROUPS, *see* Four food groups

FOOD LABELS, *see* Nutrition labeling

FOOD POISONING is really an inaccurate term. A more correct term would be *food-borne disease*. This disease or illness caused by eating the food can be the result of bacteria or a parasite in the food or the food may be contaminated by a pesticide, pollutant or dangerous metal like mercury. The symptoms of most food poisoning resemble the flu, therefore many cases are self-limiting and the person never goes to the doctor. Millions of people have a bout with food poisoning every year. For some, the elderly, infants and young children, some of these cases can lead to serious illness and even death.

If you ever suspect that you have food poisoning, here are some tips to follow:

- Treat the symptoms as you would treat the flu, making sure to take plenty of fluid to replace those lost through vomiting and diarrhea.
- If symptoms are severe or last more than a day, contact the doctor. For the elderly, infants and young children the doctor should be contacted immediately.
- Wrap up the suspect food and take it with you to the doctor or hospital.
- Contact your local Department of Health if you ate the food at a large gathering or a restaurant, or if you bought the food in a store.

There are many basic precautions that we can take to *prevent* food-borne illness:

- *Never* buy discolored, smelly, damaged food. Never taste such food!
- Cook foods thoroughly.
- Never leave foods without refrigeration for longer than two hours.
- Reheat leftovers thoroughly.
- When shopping, buy perishable items—ice cream, milk, meat—last and put away first when you get home.
- Never thaw foods on the kitchen counter; thaw in the refrigerator or microwave oven.
- Refrigerate leftovers promptly; don't cool on the kitchen counter.
- Wash your hands before handling food.
- Keep the kitchen and utensils clean.
- Do not stuff poultry.

See Vomiting, Diarrhea

FORTIFIED refers to the addition of a nutrient or nutrients to a food in amounts larger than might be found naturally or to the addition of a nutrient to a food that is not naturally found in that food. For example, milk is fortified with vitamin D and salt is fortified with iodine. Fortified is often used synonymously with "enriched," but technically these two words do not mean the same thing.

See Enriched

FOUR FOOD GROUPS separates food into four categories—milk and milk products, meat and meat substitutes, fruits and vegetables, and grains. As the foundation of an adequate diet, an adult should select a

Suggested Daily Servings from the Four Food Groups

Food Group	Recommended Number of Servings Daily For Adults	Serving Size
Milk and milk products	2*	1 cup milk 1 cup yogurt Calcium equivalents 1½ slices or 1½ ounces cheese 1 cup pudding or custard 1¾ cups ice cream 2 cups cottage cheese
Meat and meat substitutes	2	2 ounces cooked, lean meat, fish or poultry Protein equivalents 2 eggs

Food Group	Recommended Number of Servings Daily For Adults	Serving Size
		2 slices or 2 ounces cheese**
		½ cup cottage cheese**
		1 cup dried peas and beans
		¼ cup peanut butter
		6 ounces tofu (soybean curd)
Fruits and vegetables***	4 or more****	1 medium-sized fruit or vegetable
		½ cup cooked
		½ cup juice
		2 tablespoons dried fruit
Grains*****	4 or more****	1 slice bread
		1 cup cold cereal
		½ cup cooked cereal
		½ cup rice, pasta or noodles

* Children up to age nine should get 2–3 servings daily; from 9 to 12 years old 3–4 servings; 4 servings daily for teenagers, pregnant and breast-feeding women.
** Count cheese as a serving of milk *or* meat, not both simultaneously.
*** Daily choose one serving rich in vitamin C; every other day choose one serving rich in vitamin A.
**** Additional servings can be added to meet the needs of an individual's size or activity level.
***** Use whole grain or enriched products.

2-2-4-4 pattern each day: two servings from the milk group, two from the meat group, four from the fruit/vegetable group and four from the grain group. This pattern provides an adequate intake of several important nutrients and an approximate caloric intake of 1,200 Calories. Two servings from the milk or milk products group provide some protein and most of the calcium needed by an adult in a day. Two servings from the meat or meat substitute group provide adequate protein and make a substantial contribution to the daily need for iron. Four servings of fruits and vegetables will offer a wide variety of vitamins and minerals. These three groups further contribute B vitamins. Four servings of grain products (breads and cereals) provide additional B vitamins and iron. The following chart gives the minimum suggested servings from each of the four food groups.

FRUCTOSE, or fruit sugar, is a simple sugar (6 carbons) found in many fruits and honey. It is one and one half times as sweet as sugar so that smaller amounts with fewer calories can be used to provide desired sweetness.

Fructose has been shown to speed up alcohol metabolism in some persons more than others. Fructose has been suggested for use as a sweetener for diabetics because it does not have as great an effect on blood sugar levels as sucrose and it does not require the hormone insulin for absorption. Studies have shown that fructose is slightly less likely than sugar to cause cavities. Excess use of fructose can cause diarrhea.

See Carbohydrates.

FRUITS are succulent, fleshy foods that by botanical definition are the ripened ovary of a female flower from a plant. The use of fruits dates back to the beginning of human existence. The Bible says Eve tempted Adam with an apple. Figs, grapes and dates were grown in the Near East as far back as 4,000 B.C. The fruits were made into wine and dried for use during the winter. The Greeks did not use many fruits as food, believing that they would shorten life and that they caused diarrhea. Voyages by the Spanish, Portuguese, British, French and Dutch between the fifteenth and eighteenth centuries helped to exchange and distribute fruits throughout the New World and the Old World.

Fruit	Place of Origin
Apple	Caucasus Mountains of western Asia or in eastern Europe
Apricot	China
Avocado	Central America
Banana	Malay penninsula over 4,000 years ago
Blueberry	North America
Cherry	Asia
Citrus fruits (grapefruit, lemon, oragne, lime and tangerine)	Southeast Asia
Cranberry	Europe and North America
Dates	Western Asia and the Middle East
Grapes	Western Asia
Guava	American tropics
Kiwi fruit	China
Mango	India
Peach and nectarine	China
Pear	Western Asia
Persimmon	China and Japan
Pineapple	Brazil
Sapodilla	Mexico and Central America
Strawberry	Europe, North and South America
Watermelon	Africa

Fruit consumption has increased steadily in the United States during the twentieth century. Currently, we consume over 225 pounds per person a year as fresh fruit, juice, dried fruit, canned and frozen fruits. New, exotic fruits are continuously being introduced and grown successfully in many areas. For example, within the last ten years the "Chinese gooseberry," better known as *kiwi fruit,* has traveled from the Orient to Australia to California. An exotic fruit not long ago, it is fairly commonplace today, sold in supermarkets and seen regularly in recipes.

Fresh fruits are high in water and low in calories; they offer a good source of fiber and are often rich in vitamin C, as well as other essential vitamins and minerals.

Interestingly, many of the fruits commonly eaten in the United States did not originate on this continent. Following is a list of common fruits and their place of origin.

FUNGI are plants such as molds, mushrooms, toadstools and yeasts that do not contain chlorophyll, flowers or leaves. They get their nourishment by growing on living or dead organic matter.

See Brewer's yeast, Mushrooms, Yeast

G

GALLSTONES (cholelithiasis) are gravel or stones that form in the gallbladder when substances that normally are dissolved in bile precipitate out. The gallbladder stores bile made in liver that is used in fat digestion. Gallstones usually are a combination of cholesterol and bile salts and sometimes bile pigments. It is estimated that 12 million women and 4 million men in the United States are affected. People may be unaware that they have gallstones until one gets lodged in the bile duct, causing a painful attack.

Gallstones form when the gallbladder does not work properly. High fat foods, overweight, estrogens, many pregnancies, aging and low HDL levels increase the likelihood of forming gallstones.

Gallstones are treated by surgery or dissolved with drugs. A low-fat diet is used to relieve symptoms. Some sufferers find it difficult to tolerate spicy foods and gas-forming vegetables like onions, cabbage and cucumbers.

After surgery a low-fat diet is used for several weeks or months until the bile duct dilates and takes over the gallbladder function. At this time a regular diet can be resumed.

GARLIC, a plant enjoyed by some, but not all, is becoming more popular as a seasoning. Garlic bulbs were used medicinally in India in the sixth century B.C. Throughout history they were used to treat deafness, edema, lack of appetite, leprosy, parasites and other ailments. Garlic was also considered useful in keeping vampires away.

Garlic water (mashed garlic mixed into water) and garlic pills are often used as a folk remedy to reduce blood pressure. It may not be as farfetched as it sounds because studies show that garlic may reduce clogged arteries which are a factor in high blood pressure. Recent studies showed that essential oil of garlic can reduce blood cholesterol, triglycerides and low density lipoproteins (LDL) and also increase high density lipoproteins (HDL). These are all positive changes to reduce risk of coronary artery disease. For this effect one must eat about twenty raw, medium-sized cloves a day for eight months. The allicin in garlic has also been shown to kill certain types of bacteria so that it may be useful for this.

A head of garlic with 65 Calories, contains 3 gm of protein, 16 mg of calcium, 264 mg of potassium, no fat and very little sodium. When baked with the peel on, it becomes delightfully mild and delicious. Try it!

GAS (flatulence) refers to excess gas in the stomach and intestines that causes pain, bloating or gurgling. We all produce gas, some more, some less. Fortunate people expel it as it is produced so that it does not make them uncomfortable. Gas is made up mostly of hydrogen, nitrogen, methane and carbon dioxide; it contains little oxygen.

Swallowed air contributes to flatulence. Everyone swallows some air when they eat or drink. Nervous people or mouth breathers may swallow more than the usual amount. Eating slowly with mouth closed will reduce the amount of air swallowed. Chewing gum increases the amount of air swallowed as does drinking carbonated beverages. Drinking through a straw rather than gulping liquids may help. Swallowed air is expelled by belching (burping).

Gas is also produced when bacteria in the intestine ferment the undigested food residue. Some foods, like beans, have a reputation for being gas producers. The reputation is well deserved; beans contain some natural sugars that are hard to digest, so they ferment in the intestine. Different kinds of beans produce varying amounts of gas. Baked beans have been shown to increase gas output ten times over the normal level. Soaking dry beans and discarding the water, then using fresh water to cook them for thirty minutes and then again discarding this water and finishing the cooking with fresh water has been shown to reduce the gas-forming potential of beans.

Other foods, such as onions, celery, carrots, raisins, broccoli, cabbage, cauliflower, bananas, apricots, prune juice, pretzels, bagels, cucumber, radishes, wheat germ and brussels sprouts, also promote gas formation in some people. Even applesauce has been shown to cause gas.

Lactose intolerance, the inability to digest lactose (milk sugar) completely, can be another cause of excess gas. The addition of brewer's yeast or of fiber-containing foods like whole wheat and bran can also cause more gas than usual. It usually takes about three weeks to adjust to the change in diet.

Because there are so many foods that produce excess gas, it is helpful to keep a diary recording everything eaten and gassy episodes; it will show the connection between gas produced after specific foods are eaten. Foods that should be reduced or eliminated will become evident.

See Lactose intolerance

GASTRIC is a term pertaining to the stomach.

GASTRIC STAPLING or gastroplasty is a reduction in the capacity of the stomach resulting from physical division of the stomach cavity by stapling off a portion of the stomach. It causes weight loss by reducing food intake and delaying the emptying of the stomach, and is used for people who are two or three times normal weight. Complications are less serious than for intestinal bypass surgery, another drastic treatment for extreme obesity. As gastric stapling is a fairly new procedure, its long-term effects have not yet been evaluated.

GATORADE is a sports drink called a sweat replacer. It contains water, glucose, syrup solids, sucrose, citric acid, natural lemon and lime flavors, salt, sodium citrate, monopotassium phosphate, ester gum and Yellow #5. An 8-ounce serving provides 50 Calories, 14 gm carbohydrate, 110 mg of sodium, 25 mg of potassium and no protein or fat.

See Sports drinks

GELATIN is a mixture of protein made from bones, skin, tendons and ligaments of animals. It is often used as a food additive in candy and ice cream and as the basis for molded desserts and salads. Gelatin has a reputation for strengthening brittle nails and hair. The basis for this claim is that hair and nails are made of protein so an additional source of protein should improve their condition. This is not true.

Although gelatin is a protein, it does not contain all the needed amino acids so it must be supplemented with other protein before it can be used to build body tissue. Besides this, growth and appearance of hair and nails would be affected only when the food intake is very deficient and that would cause other body symptoms as well. In short, brittle nails and hair will not be improved by eating gelatin.

See Amino acids, Protein

GEOPHAGIA is eating clay or earth. Excessive clay eating can cause reduced absorption and deficiency of minerals.

See Pica

GERIATRICS is the medical specialty dealing with the prevention and treatment of diseases of aging. It is one area in the field of *gerontology,* which covers all aspects of aging.

There are no special food or nutrient supplements that are best for all the elderly. Needs should be determined individually for each person.

There has not been enough research to determine exactly what are the nutritional needs at this time of life. What is known is that the need for Calories generally decreases as people age while the need for protein, vitamins and minerals remains the same or may be increased.

GINSENG has been used, mainly in China, for thousands of years as a health tonic, stimulant and aphrodisiac. In the United States it is estimated that 5 to 6 million people use it. Ginseng can be purchased in liquid, powder or capsule form and it is often brewed into tea. It has been advertised as guaranteeing a joyful temper, plenty of pure red blood and relief from irritable bladder.

Ginseng is classified pharmacologically as an *adaptogen* because experimental studies suggest that it may help the body *adapt* to stress and correct adrenal and thyroid dysfunction. Ginseng is often recommended during menopause. Research supporting this is inconclusive.

Occasional use of ginseng may be helpful and probably would cause no harm. Many products like teas and tonics contain mainly milk sugar (lactose) and very little ginseng, but doses as low as 0.5 gram have been reported therapeutically effective. Daily use of high doses, 3 grams or more daily, may be harmful. Some ginseng users developed high blood pressure, nervousness, sleeplessness, skin eruptions and morning diarrhea with use at this level.

GLUCOMANNON is a fiber (nondigestable substance) that is obtained from Konjac tubers grown originally in Japan. It has been recommended as an aid to weight control and is sold in wafers and capsules. Glucomannon absorbs water and swells up filling the stomach so that less food is eaten.

Emergency medical treatment has been needed to remove swollen glucomannon tablets that became lodged in the throats of persons who had taken the preparation and tried to wash it down with water.

GLUCOSE, or dextrose, is a simple sugar (6 carbons). Three-fourths as sweet as sugar, it is formed in the body from starch as it is digested. In the body all other sugars and starches are eventually converted into glucose. Glucose is the sugar circulating in the blood that provides the body's major source of energy. Intravenous solutions contain glucose usually at the 5 percent level (D_5W). Corn syrup is mainly glucose; grapes, berries, oranges and carrots also contain some glucose.

See Carbohydrate

GLUCOSE TOLERANCE FACTOR (GTF) is a hormonelike substance that contains chromium and niacin (a B vitamin) along with protein. This factor helps the body use glucose (carbohydrate) normally, by increasing the activity of the hormone insulin. Some people with diabetes who were deficient in chromium inproved their ability to use glucose after they were given chromium supplements. That does not mean that they were cured, only that their condition was made less severe. Persons with normal chromium levels in their body will not benefit from additional supplements.

The glucose tolerance factor sold in health food stores is derived from yeast.

GLUCOSE TOLERANCE TEST measures blood glucose (sugar) levels after a dose of glucose is given. This determines the rate of glucose uptake from the blood by body cells. Removal of glucose from the blood is largely dependent on insulin levels.

Prior to the test, the person should be eating a normal amount of carbohydrate, at least 150 grams a day. The person drinks a cola or lemon-flavored beverage containing 75 to 100 grams of glucose and the blood sugar levels are measured at hour intervals for up to five hours. Increased levels of blood glucose and a delayed return to normal values along with abnormally low blood glucose levels occurring in three to five hours may indicate diabetes. Many drugs and other illnesses can also affect blood glucose levels.

A blood glucose level of 40 to 60 mg/dl at three hours may indicate hypoglycemia or low blood sugar.

See Diabetes, Blood sugar, Hypoglycemia

GLYCOGEN (animal starch) is the main form of carbohydrate (glucose) stored in the body. It is found in the liver and in muscles where it is a ready source of energy. Glycogen helps sustain normal blood sugar levels during sleep and during fasting. Compared to fat, very little energy is stored as glycogen.

See Carbohydrate, Glycogen loading

GLYCOGEN LOADING, also known as carbohydrate loading, refers to a combination of diet and exercise which can result in the muscles storing two or three times more glycogen than normal. Glycogen, a stored carbohydrate, is an important source of energy for muscles. This loading provides greater energy reserves and can be of value to the athlete who participates in long distance or extended activities.

Glycogen loading is started one week before the event. On the first day exhausting exercise is done to deplete the glycogen stores in specific muscles. On the second, third and fourth days a low-carbohydrate diet is eaten along with exercise. On the fifth, sixth and seventh days high carbohydrate foods (rice, pasta, potatoes, lentils, breads) are incorporated into the diet. During these three days, exercise is decreased so that glycogen is retained in the muscles.

This causes a temporary increase in weight as water (which is heavy) is stored with the glycogen—approximately 3 grams of water to 1 gram of glycogen. Some athletes complain that this makes their muscles feel waterlogged, stiff and not as responsive.

Glycogen loading may be harmful. There have been reports of resulting heart irregularities. It may also be harmful to persons susceptible to diabetes, kidney or heart disease. Growing athletes should never practice glycogen loading. It may be safer and simpler to increase carbohydrate stores by resting and eating a lot of carbohydrates for a few days before the athletic event.

See Sports nutrition

GOITER is an enlargement of the thyroid gland in the neck. It is usually the result of an iodine (mineral) deficiency, although it may have other causes. The thyroid gland swells in an attempt to produce more hormone. Goiter is more common in females than in males and is most likely to develop during puberty or pregnancy when there is a greater need for thyroid hormones. At one time goiter was prevalent in persons living in the Great Lakes region. Iodine was added to salt in an attempt to combat this deficiency disease.

At the present time the iodine intake of Americans averages three to four times the RDA, most of it coming from dairy products, food colors and sanitizing agents used in food processing. Excess iodine consumption can cause goiter just as iodine deficiency can.

See Iodine

GOITROGENS are substances that produce goiters when they are eaten. Members of the cabbage family—kohlrabi, mustard greens, cabbage, turnips, brussels sprouts, cauliflower, rutabaga, kale and soybean products—contain goitrogens but they may be inactivated during cooking. These goitrogens act on the thyroid gland to prevent it from making thyroid hormone. Large amounts may interfere with thyroid medication (Synthroid) so that persons taking this drug should eat only moderate amounts of these vegetables.

See Goiter

GOUT is an inborn error of uric acid metabolism that doesn't appear till adulthood when it causes arthritislike symptoms. Men, who have gout more often than women, show signs of the problem around age 35. The rare woman with gout usually will not show symptoms until after menopause.

With gout a person cannot eliminate uric acid from the body efficiently; the acid builds up and deposits form in small joints and surrounding tissue. The toes, particularly the large toe, become painful and the pain may radiate up the leg. Gout can be treated with drugs that regulate the uric acid level. Dietary treatment is less important, however, a diet low in fat, high in carbohydrate and moderate in protein will help the drug control the uric acid level. Overeating, alcohol, fasting, diuretics (water pills) and overweight all can aggravate gout causing more frequent, painful attacks. Anchovies, gravies, broth, liver, herring, mussels, scallops and brewer's yeast produce large amounts of uric acid when metabolized in the body. Persons with gout should limit their use of these foods. Drinking plenty of water will help eliminate uric acid.

See Arthritis

GRAHAM CRACKERS, made from finely ground whole wheat flour, are the legacy of an early food faddist, Sylvester Graham. He believed indigestion was the result of too concentrated a diet and the way to cure it was to put bran back into white flour. Graham, born in 1794, and his converts Grahamites, preached abstinence from meat and increased use of whole wheat for both physical and spiritual reasons. Before his death at 57, he lectured at leading universities, set up Graham boardinghouses serving healthy vegetarian fare, and organized Graham teas for ladies "to discuss intimate female problems over bran tea and Graham milk toast." These may have been the first consciousness-raising sessions. Some credit Sylvester Graham with being the "father of public health."

GRAINS, *see* cereals

GRANOLA, as originally formulated, was a mixture

of rolled oats, wheat germ, sea salt, sesame seeds, coconut, brown sugar and soy oil sold as a so-called "health food" cereal. There are now many variations of granola available as cereals and snacks which contain some or all of the above ingredients along with honey, nuts, spices or fruit. These granola products are often high in fat and sugar and therefore higher in calories than many other cereals. Compare, for example, the following two products:

<u>Nature Valley Fruit and Nut Granola (General Mills)—</u>
1 ounce
128 Calories
4.0 gm fat
20.7 gm carbohydrate (29 percent sugar)
3.0 gm protein

<u>Corn Flakes (Kelloggs)—1 ounce</u>
109 Calories
0.0 fat
19 gm carbohydrate (5 percent sugar)
1.5 gm protein

GRAPEFRUIT DIET, *see* Diet

GRAS stands for "generally recognized as safe." When the Food Additives Amendment was added to the Federal Food, Drug and Cosmetic Act in 1958, some items were exempted from the testing requirements because they were judged by experts to be "generally recognized as safe" under the conditions of their use at that time.

In 1980 the government concluded an extensive re-evaluation of additives currently in use. Of the 415 substances on the GRAS list at that time, 305 retained their safe status. Those items that were removed from the GRAS list will be regulated under another category for additive use. They may be returned to the GRAS list once required testing is completed and they are again determined to be safe as used. Currently the Food and Drug Administration is implementing new regulations for GRAS additives to ensure increased safety in our food supply.

See Additives

H

HAIR ANALYSIS has been promoted as a way of diagnosing vitamin and mineral deficiencies. Minerals can be measured in hair, but vitamins cannot; they break down in the hair as its cells die.

Scientists are not sure that hair levels of minerals reflect blood levels of these substances. Hair can be contaminated with shampoos, conditioners, water, dyes and air pollution that can give false readings. Red hair naturally contains more iron than other hair colors. Even if the mineral levels were accurate, there are no standard lab values to measure them against.

Mail order hair analysis companies have been known to diagnose conditions that don't exist, provide differing analysis for the same hair sample at different times and suggest the use of many supplements that they are ready to sell.

Hair analysis is useful under certain conditions. It can show if a person died from arsenic or lead poisoning. It has also been used to compare mineral levels in groups of people living in different parts of the country. This can help point out areas where there is contamination in the water or soil depletion.

HDL is an abbreviation for high density lipoprotein.

See Lipoprotein

HEALTH FOODS are foods that are said to improve health, prevent disease or even cure disease. Foods called "natural" or "organic" fall under the umbrella of so-called *health food*. So do such foods as wheat germ, sprouts, rose hips, fertile eggs, sunflower seeds, sea salt, honey and yogurt. While there is nothing wrong with eating these foods, it is unrealistic to expect unusual benefits from them. "Health foods" do not necessarily promote good health. Some of them are safe and are beneficial as part of a diet; others are unnecessary, costly or even harmful. According to a 1978 ruling of the Federal Trade Commission, the term "health food" can be used in a store name but it cannot be used in food advertising or labeling because it may falsely attribute special or superior properties to certain foods.

Most industry and United States Department of Agriculture (USDA) officials agree on proper use of the term "natural." These foods cannot contain artificial or synthetic ingredients and can only be "minimally processed." Minimal processing includes canning, bottling or freezing, baking, roasting, grinding and other techniques that can be done in a home kitchen. In 1978, the Federal Trade Commission (FTC) proposed that this guideline serve as a legal definition of "natural" but it was not formally adopted. Since 1981 the USDA has used that definition in labeling meat and poultry products.

Natural does not always equal good nutrition, as many foods, such as potato chips, qualify as natural as long as the manufacturer fully discloses the ingredients. Vinegar is just as natural as it always was, the only difference is that some brands now use the word "natural" on the label.

Organic foods refer to crops grown using only natural fertilizers or composts but no chemical pesticides, herbicides, fertilizers or synthetic additives. Animals must be fed organically grown rations and no growth regulators.

Only three states—California, Oregon and Maine—have established standards for foods that are advertised or labeled "organic." Studies have shown more "organic" produce is sold than is actually grown.

HEART ATTACK is caused by reduced blood flow to the heart muscle. The reduced blood flow is caused by a stopped-up (occluded) artery (atherosclerosis). Symptoms are often severe pain in chest, shoulder and arm along with shortness of breath. Some people have "silent attacks" they are not aware of.

Myocardial infarct (MI) is the medical term for heart attack. Attacks are most likely to occur between 6 and 9 A.M.

HEARTBURN is a burning sensation felt in the area of the throat and heart that actually has nothing to do with the heart. It is caused by a reflux (regurgitation) of food and acid from the stomach into the esophagus, the tube that carries food from the mouth to the stomach. The backing-up of stomach contents irritates the esophagus, causing a burning sensation. Sometimes the food and acid pass all the way up to the mouth.

A too full stomach can be the cause of heartburn. Another cause is a relaxed lower esophageal sphincter (LES), the muscle around the opening between the esophagus and stomach. The LES can be relaxed from regular and decaffeinated coffee, chocolate, alcohol, food high in fat, peppermint and spearmint flavorings. Smoking cigarettes relaxes the muscle as well. Skim milk has the opposite effect and may be helpful.

Extra fat on the belly, lying down, lifting something

heavy or bending over can start the backing-up process that results in heartburn.

Eating three small meals a day with a mid-morning and mid-afternoon snack, avoiding food in the two hours before bedtime and drinking liquids between meals rather than with them all may help avoid heartburn. Heartburn may also be a symptom of hiatus hernia.

See Hiatus hernia

HEIGHT-WEIGHT TABLES are usually based on material published by the Metropolitan Life Insurance Company that has been obtained from life expectancy data of owners of life insurance. They may not actually be representative of all Americans and the weights should not be considered a precise standard or weight goal but rather a guide. The Tables were last revised in 1983.

See Body frame

Metropolitan Insurance Companies

1983 Metropolitan Height and Weight Tables

MEN

Height Feet inches	Small Frame	Medium Frame	Large Frame
5 2	128–134	131–141	138–150
5 3	130–136	133–143	140–153
5 4	132–138	135–145	142–156
5 5	134–140	137–148	144–160
5 6	136–142	139–151	146–164
5 7	138–145	142–154	149–168
5 8	140–148	145–157	152–172
5 9	142–151	148–160	155–176
5 10	144–154	151–163	158–180
5 11	146–157	154–166	161–184
6 0	149–160	157–170	164–188
6 1	152–164	160–174	168–192
6 2	155–168	164–178	172–197
6 3	158–172	167–182	176–202
6 4	162–176	171–187	181–207

Weights at Ages 25-59 Based on Lowest Mortality. Weight in Pounds According to Frame (in indoor clothing weighing 5 lbs., shoes with 1" heels).

WOMEN

Height Feet inches	Small Frame	Medium Frame	Large Frame
4 10	102–111	109–121	118–131
4 11	103–113	111–123	120–134
5 0	104–115	113–126	122–137
5 1	106–118	115–129	125–140
5 2	108–121	118–132	128–143
5 3	111–124	121–135	131–147
5 4	114–127	124–138	134–151
5 5	117–130	127–141	137–155
5 6	120–133	130–144	140–159
5 7	123–136	133–147	143–163
5 8	126–139	136–150	146–167
5 9	129–142	139–153	149–170
5 10	132–145	142–156	152–173
5 11	135–148	145–159	155–176
6 0	138–151	148–162	158–179

Weights at Ages 25-59 Based on Lowest Mortality. Weight in Pounds According to Frame (in indoor clothing weighing 3 lbs., shoes with 1" heels).

HEMATOCRIT (Hct) is the percentage of whole blood volume occupied by red cells after the blood is centrifuged (spun to separate the solid from the liquid portion). It is also called packed cell volume. It is measured as milliliters per deciliter (ml/dl).

NORMAL HEMATOCRIT VALUES
Men	40–54 ml/dl
Women	37–47 ml/dl
Children	36–40 ml/dl

Low values may point to anemia due to deficiency of iron, folic acid or vitamin B_{12}.

See Hemoglobin

HEMOGLOBIN (Hg, Hgb) is the iron containing pigment-protein compound that gives color to red blood cells and carries oxygen in the blood. It is measured in grams per deciliter (g/dl) in the blood.

NORMAL HEMOGLOBIN VALUES
Women	12.6–14.2 g/dl
Men	14.0–16.5 g/dl
Children	12.0–14.0 g/dl

Lower levels may indicate anemia.

In pregnancy, normal level is over 10.6 g/dl. At all ages, in both sexes blacks have hemoglobin levels of about .5 g lower.

See Hematocrit

HERBAL TEA is a beverage resulting when hot water and an herb or spice are allowed to steep so that volatile flavors and fragrances leach from the plant into the water. Almost any herb or spice or combination can be brewed into a tea. The Food and Drug Administration considers herbal teas as beverages and simply requires that they be labeled correctly with contents disclosed. If the tea is mixed and sold locally these regulations do not apply.

An occasional cup of herbal tea is warming, pleasant and fragrant. There are instances, however, when excessive use of herbal teas may prove harmful. Some herbs, like buckthorn bark, senna, dock root, aloe, fo-ti and poke root may cause diarrhea. Others, such as pennyroyal, blue cohosh, comfrey, rue and tansy may be harmful during pregnancy or lactation. For people with allergies, flower teas like chamomile or yarrow may cause a reaction. Health Inca Tea (HIT) and Mate de Coca tea contain detectable levels of cocaine which produce mild stimulation, mood elevation and increased pulse rate. When trying a new variety of herbal tea, select those that have accurate labeling, make a weak brew at first and do not drink many cups at one time.

Herbal teas that have been shown to be safe are: Red Zinger, lemon balm, rose hip, raspberry, lemon grass and mint tea.

See Herbs

HERBS are plants or parts of plants valued for their savory, aromatic or medicinal qualities. Some herbs are used to flavor foods, others give a scent and some have medicinal qualities. Many of our modern medicines originated as herbal remedies—digitalis comes from foxglove, poppies are made into morphine and aloe vera soothes burns.

Currently there has been a resurgence of interest in herbs, both as foods and as medicines. In most cases, used in moderation herbs are harmless. Some, however, have potential harmful effects. Herbs are neither classified as a food, nor a drug so that the Food and Drug Administration (FDA) has limited regulatory power over their sale or use. The FDA can take action only after it receives a report of a serious health risk

Potentially Dangerous Herbs

Herb	Health Claims	Part Used
Angelica	breaks up gas, brings on menstruation	root, leaves and fruit
Blue cohosh	causes uterine contractions, brings on menstruation	rootstem, root
Broom	mind-altering (when smoked)	flowering top
Calamus	lowers fever, helps digestion	rootstem
Canaigre	tonic	root
Chaparral	restores healthy body function, anti-cancer	leaves, twigs
Coltsfoot	cough medicine, soothing gummy or oily ointment	leaves, flower heads
Comfrey	general healing agent	rootstem, roots, leaves
Dong quai	uterine tonic, relieves spasms, restores healthy body function	root
Eyebright	treats eye diseases, conjunctivitis	entire plant above ground
Life root	brings on menstruation, treats uterine diseases	entire plant
Mistletoe	increases blood pressure, relieves spasms, reduces blood pressure	leaves
Pennyroyal	causes abortion, brings on menstruation	leaves, oil
Pokeweed	restores healthy	root

Herb	Health Claims	Part Used
	body function, relieves rheumatism, anticancer, stimulates bowel movement	
Sassafras	stimulant, relieves spasms, causes sweating, relieves rheumatism, tonic	root bark
Wormwood	cures worms, tonic, mind-altering	leaves, tops

from using an herbal. For example, the FDA banned the use of safrole, a part of sassafras, and sassafras oil in 1960 because these substances were found to be carcinogenic (cancer-causing).

Although herbs are natural they may still contain powerful chemicals in unknown quantities. They react more like drugs than foods. Following are some suggestions to consider before using an herbal remedy.

- *Use only a small amount*. Use one-quarter to one-fifth of the suggested dose to minimize any harmful reaction.
- *Don't use the oil of herbs*. They are more potent and even small doses can be harmful.
- *Don't harvest herbs from unknown sources*. Roadside harvesting could result in eating a lead- or pesticide-contaminated herb. There is also the possibility of harvesting a look-alike that could be poisonous.
- *Use only those herbs known to be safe*. The local poison control center can provide guidance.
- *Don't substitute herbs for medical help*. Tell your doctor about the herbal remedy you intend to try; if you get sick after taking an herb, seek medical help and bring a sample of the herb with you.

- *Don't mix herbs and other medicines without checking first*. Some herbs and drugs are not compatible and can cause you harm.

See Herbal tea

HIATUS HERNIA occurs when the upper part of the stomach slides through the esophageal opening and into the chest cavity. Causes can be obesity, pregnancy, severe coughing, wearing tight clothes around the waist and weightlifting. It is estimated that half of all adults in the United States have a mild degree of hiatus hernia, but only a few have symptoms. Major symptoms are heartburn, pressure in abdomen and more rarely, the feeling of food stuck in the throat.

Losing weight is beneficial. Avoiding too much food and drink at one time, especially late in the day, which can distend the stomach is important. A diet low in fat and high in protein will help keep the food in the stomach. Enough fiber should be eaten to prevent constipation and the straining at the stools it causes. Black pepper, chili powder, coffee, cocoa, tea and alcohol are irritants and should be avoided. Lying down or exercising after meals can cause discomfort as can clothes that are tight around the waist and midriff.

In the past antacids were recommended to be taken one hour after meals and at bedtime. Recent research disputes the value of this practice.

See Heartburn, Lower esophageal sphincter

HIGH BLOOD PRESSURE, *see* Hypertension

HIGH FIBER DIET, *see* Diet

HIGH PROTEIN DIETS are often therapeutically used when stress, infection and trauma (burns, surgery, serious injury) are present. A high protein diet is planned to supply 100 to 125 gm of protein (twice the RDA) and at least 2,500 Calories. Sufficient calories are needed so that the protein is not used for energy. At least half of the protein should come from animal sources like milk, eggs and meat and should be divided among the day's meals. Nonfat dry milk can be added to liquid milk to increase the protein. Two to four tablespoons are added per cup.

High protein diets are sometimes planned as weight loss diets. In this case, the total Calorie content is low, while the protein level is high.

See Diet

HONEY is made by bees from the nectar of flowers. This pleasant tasting syrup has a reputation for being a healthier sweetener than sugar. It isn't; in fact, it is very similar to sugar and no more nutritious in spite of the fact that it does contain tiny amounts of vitamins and minerals. If you ate a whole cup of honey (1,031 Calories) you would get one half of your daily need for one vitamin, B_{12}, and far less of other nutrients.

Honey has been recommended as a cure for bedwetting, sleeplessness, migraine headaches, muscle cramps, runny noses and arthritis. There is no scientific evidence to support any of these claims.

As honey is about twice as sweet as sugar, less can be used—however, the calorie savings are slight as one tablespoon of honey contains 64 Calories, while one tablespoon of sugar has 46 Calories.

Infants less than one year old should not be fed honey. A serious form of food poisoning, infant botulism, has occurred in a few instances after honey was used. This type of botulism poisoning does not occur after infancy.

HUNGER is a physiological desire for food after a period of time has passed since food was last eaten.

Contractions of an empty stomach, "hunger pangs," develop when a person has gone a long time without food. Hunger is a short-term problem eliminated by eating. When it is prolonged, starvation and malnutrition develop.

Many of us experience hunger mid-morning if we have skipped breakfast. Adults may become grouchy and irritable. That's why you need a "coffee break." Hungry children have difficulty with school work. Research has shown that hungry children make more mistakes on tests.

HYDROGENIZATION refers to the process by which hydrogen is added to the double bonds of unsaturated fatty acids. This hardens the fat, turning liquid oil into solid fat. This more saturated fat has a higher melting point and stays fresh longer. Margarine and solid white shortenings (such as Crisco) are hydrogenated.

HYPER- is a prefix meaning above normal or an excess.

HYPERACTIVITY, *see* Feingold Diet

HYPERCHOLESTEROLEMIA is an elevation of cholesterol in the blood. There are differing opinions as to what level of cholesterol in the blood actually constitutes overt hypercholesterolemia. Some experts says that hypercholesterolemia is defined as concentrations over 260 mg/dl, which is generally accepted as the upper limit of normal for American adults. Considerable evidence, however, shows that there is a relationship between coronary heart disease incidence and cholesterol at concentrations above 230 mg/dl. Adult men can be considered mildly hypercholesterolemic at concentrations in the range of 200 to 260 mg/dl. Cholesterol levels can be lowered in many ways—weight reduction, increased exercise and through dietary changes. The American Heart Association has recommended that the daily intake of cholesterol should not be more than 300 mg per day.

See Cholesterol, Hyperlipidemia

HYPERGLYCEMIA is elevated blood sugar.

See Blood sugar

HYPERLIPIDEMIA is an elevation of one or more of the lipids (fats) in the blood. It generally refers to increased levels of cholesterol or triglycerides. Hyperlipidemia is considered a major factor in coronary heart disease.

See Cholesterol, HDL, Hypercholesterolemia, Hypertriglyceridemia, LDL

HYPERTENSION, or high blood pressure, refers to repeated blood pressure readings of 140/90 mm or above.

About one out of five people will develop high blood pressure during their lifetime. Many are unaware that they have it because there may be no symptoms. In most high blood pressure, about 90 percent of all cases, there is no single, easily identified cause. In other situations, high blood pressure can be caused by kidney ailments, endocrine gland malfunction, pregnancy or the use of oral contraceptives.

If high blood pressure is not treated, there may be damage to the kidney, eyes, brain and blood vessels. Treatment consists of weight loss if needed, salt restriction, life-style changes (exercise and relaxation) and avoiding tobacco use.

HYPERTRIGLYCERIDEMIA refers to elevated

blood levels of triglycerides. Hypertriglyceridemia is almost always an inherited disorder but it can also be caused or further aggravated by oral contraceptives, excessive caffeine intake, supplementation with vitamin A and alcohol abuse.

Evaluating plasma triglycerides is part of preventive care to determine the risk for cardiovascular disease. When the cholesterol level is normal, mild elevations of triglycerides, less than 250 mg/dl, do not predict an increased risk for heart disease. Borderline hypertriglyceridemia, 250–500 mg/dl, is only predictive of risk if there are other risk factors such as family history of heart disease, hypertension, obesity, diabetes or smoking. A person with triglycerides in this range may be in the group of people with the hereditary form of hypertriglyceridemia and they should be reevaluated on a regular basis and encouraged to watch other risk factors. True hypertriglyceridemia occurs when serum levels go above 500 mg/dl; it requires treatment. A person with very high triglyceride values should be encouraged to lose weight, increase exercise, restrict alcohol, reduce the use of sugars and other sweets, and eat a low fat diet. It takes several months to a year before these dietary and life-style changes will be reflected in the serum levels of triglycerides.

See Hypercholesterolemia, Hyperlipidemia

HYPERVITAMINOSIS, or vitamin poisoning, refers to excess intake of vitamins. This usually is the result of taking too many vitamin supplements. It is practically impossible to develop this condition from eating too much ordinary food. In 1982, the Poison Control Center estimated over thirty thousand cases of overdoses on vitamin-mineral supplements. About 5 thousand of these cases were people over 5 years old.

When more of a vitamin is taken than is needed, the excess acts like a drug in the body and may have negative side effects. The most usual vitamin poisonings that have been reported are with vitamins A and D. These vitamins dissolve in fat and can be stored in large amounts in the body, particularly the liver, and they have toxic effects. These vitamins are taken in large doses because it is believed they are effective against common problems. Vitamin A is used to treat acne; vitamin D has been used for arthritis.

Hypervitaminosis A can cause loss of appetite, dry itching skin, hair loss, swollen joints and enlarged liver.

Hypervitaminosis D can cause loss of appetite, nausea, headache, vomiting, excess urination, diarrhea, fatigue, calcium deposits in kidneys, high blood pressure and high blood cholesterol levels.

There have been reports of undesirable side effects from other vitamins—E, K, C and B vitamins—as well.

See Megadoses

HYPO-, HYP-, is a prefix meaning a deficiency or lack of a substance.

HYPOGLYCEMIA, or low blood sugar, is often blamed for a variety of symptoms like hunger, headaches, depression, phobia, anxiety, sweating and palpitations. This disorder is controversial as some experts feel it is not a true disease. Actually, these symptoms can be caused by a variety of problems so that a person experiencing them should seek a medical diagnosis. There are very few people who regularly produce too much insulin so their blood sugar is abnormally low. Such a condition can be diagnosed by a glucose tolerance test or a simple blood test at the time a person is experiencing symptoms.

Hypoglycemia is treated with frequent, small meals rich in complex carbohydrates (like beans and lentils), containing a good fiber content and few concentrated sweets.

See Carbohydrates, Glucose tolerance test

HYPO-, HYPERKALEMIA, *see* Potassium

INDIGESTION, also called dyspepsia, is a general term that covers disorders associated with eating—pain, burning, belching, bloating, nausea, gas and regurgitation of food into the mouth. Most of us are bothered with these discomforts at one time or another. Persons experiencing frequent symptoms should see a doctor to rule out any physical cause. In most cases indigestion is due to tension or to an intolerance to certain food.

Alcohol, coffee, tea, cola, pepper, chili powder and foods high in protein increase the production of stomach acid. Elimination or reduction of these spices and drinks and eating high protein foods along with other foods can help.

How often and where you eat may be even more important than what is eaten:

- Eat meals at regular times and never overeat.
- Eat three small meals daily supplemented by two snacks, mid-morning and mid-afternoon.
- Take meals and snacks in a pleasant, peaceful environment.
- Eat slowly and calmly.

See Antacids

INFANT FORMULA, available in powdered or liquid form, is usually cow's milk that has been modified so that it is more like human breast milk. The protein and mineral content is reduced while the carbohydrate (sugar) is increased, and vegetable oil replaces the butterfat. As more information is learned about breast milk, formulas are changed. Infants fed formula grow just as well as if breast-fed. The disadvantages are that formula-fed babies have more allergies, constipation, diarrhea and gastrointestinal and respiratory infections. There is a greater chance that formula-fed babies may be fed too much and become overweight, perhaps because it is easy to see when some formula remains in the bottle—the baby may be urged to finish it all. Another disadvantage is that care must be taken to prepare or dilute the formula properly unless it is purchased ready to use. If water is used to prepare formula, it should be safe to drink. Unused formula must be refrigerated or discarded.

When an infant is shown to be allergic to cow's milk, a specialized formula can be substituted.

INFECTION occurs when the body is invaded by disease-producing bacteria. When an infection develops, body cells make antibodies to combat the infection. Nutritional deficiency can reduce resistance to infection and infection increases the body's need for nutrients. The body reacts to the stress of infection by losing nutrients, especially protein and minerals. Vomiting and diarrhea and increased perspiration add to water losses; fever does as well. At the same time a fever will increase the body's use of calories.

See Diarrhea, Fever, Vomiting

INOSITOL is an alcohol, related in structure to 6 carbon sugars. It is found in many foods particularly in cereal bran. It is an essential nutrient for mice and rats, but has not as yet been found to be essential for humans.

INSULIN is a hormone secreted by the beta cells of the islets of the pancreas. It helps regulate the metabolism of carbohydrate and fat. Its main role may be to help glucose get into body cells. A deficiency of insulin causes diabetes, more precisely called diabetes mellitus. In diabetes there is an elevation of blood sugar (glucose) levels. About 25 percent of all people with diabetes are given insulin. As insulin is a protein it is digested if taken by mouth so it must be given by injection.

In the past insulin was used to increase the appetite. It is rarely used for this purpose now.

See Diabetes

INTESTINAL IMPACTIONS, or bezoars, are tightly packed masses of hair, fruit or vegetable fibers that can become stuck in the intestine. These obstructions are usually made up of pulp, seeds, husks and skins of fruits and vegetables. Oranges, persimmons, potato skins and unshelled pumpkin seeds, when eaten in large amounts, can cause the problem. Pain, feeling full, nausea, vomiting and constipation may be symptoms of an impaction. People of all ages can develop bezoars but they are found most often in those over 60. Loss of teeth, chewing problems and difficulties with emptying the stomach can set the stage for intestinal impactions. They are treated with enzyme preparations or surgical removal.

INTRINSIC FACTOR, see Vitamin B_{12}

IODINE is an essential mineral found in the body in small amounts. The body contains about 25 mg of iodine; almost half of it is in the thyroid gland. It is used to make thyroid hormones that control the metabolic rate. A deficiency of iodine can cause enlargement of the thyroid gland called *goiter*. The gland swells to make up for the lack of iodine. A more serious disorder, *cretinism*, can occur in babies born to women severely deficient in iodine. Babies with cretinism are retarded mentally and physically.

Iodine deficiencies can occur when most food eaten is grown on soils that contain low levels of the mineral. To avoid this possibility in the United States, iodine is added to salt; it is said to be *iodized*. This is voluntary but it is estimated that more than one half of salt is iodized.

Iodine is also found in seafood and seaweeds like kelp. Vegetables, milk and eggs may also be good sources if the soils contain sufficient iodine and if the cows and chickens get iodine-supplemented feed.

The RDA for iodine is 150 mcg for adults. Studies have shown that we get about four times this amount, most of it from dairy products due to sanitizers (iodophors) used to clean dairying equipment. Food colors, dough conditioners used in baked goods and pollutants are also sources. Long term, excessive iodine intake can disturb the function of the thyroid gland and also lead to goiter. Some experts say that iodized salt may no longer be needed.

See Goiter

IRON is an essential mineral found in the body in small amounts—only 3 to 4 gm in an adult. Seventy percent of this iron is part of hemoglobin, the pigment in red blood cells that carries oxygen throughout the body. The rest of the iron is in enzymes or is stored as reserve in the liver, spleen and bone marrow.

Iron in foods is not absorbed very well. A greater

percentage is absorbed from meat and less is absorbed from vegetables and cereals. Vitamin C and the eating of meat, fish or poultry at a meal will increase the total amount of iron absorbed. When the body has a greater need for iron during growth, pregnancy and blood losses, absorption is increased. Surgical removal of the stomach and taking in excess amounts of *phytates* from grains, *oxylates* from spinach and chocolate, and *tannins* from tea all can reduce iron absorption.

Iron in Foods

Food	Portion	Milligrams of iron
Apple	1 medium	0.5
Apricots, dried	4 halves	0.8
Avocado	½	1.3
Bean sprouts	½ cup	0.5
Beef	3 ounces	2.7
Blueberries	⅝ cup	1.0
Bread, white	1 slice	0.6
Bread, whole-wheat	1 slice	0.8
Chickpeas	½ cup	3.0
Corn muffin	1	0.6
Egg	1	1.1
Chicken, fried	¼	1.8
Grape-nuts	1 ounce	0.5
Green beans	½ cup	0.4
Kidney beans	½ cup	2.2
Liver	3 ounces	8.0
Molasses	1 tablespoon	0.9
Peanuts, roasted	1 tablespoon	0.5
Potato	1 small	0.5
Prunes	4	1.5
Prune juice	½ cup	5.2
Raisins	1 tablespoon	0.4
Split peas, dried	½ cup	1.5
Turkey	3 ounces	1.5
Walnuts	1 tablespoon	0.2

A deficiency of iron can cause iron-deficiency anemia with symptoms of weakness, pale skin and mucous membranes, fatigue, rapid heartbeat, shortness of breath, sore tongue and tingling of fingers and toes. A deficiency is more likely during adolescence (in girls especially), in pregnancy, when children grow rapidly, and in infancy when babies are born with low iron reserves or when their diet is inadequate.

The RDA for iron is 18 mg for women up to age fifty-one and 10 mg for women over age fifty-one and for all adult males. The RDA for children ranges from 10 mg for infants up to six months to 18 mg for older children and female adolescents. Good food sources are meats, especially organ meats like liver, poultry, fish, enriched and whole grain breads and cereals, dried peas and beans, eggs, dried apricots and prunes.

See Anemia, Minerals

IRRADIATION, approved for use in twenty-eight countries, may soon become important as a food processing technique in the United States. Food is irradiated or picowaved by the use of ionizing radiation from radioactive isotopes such as cobalt or cesium or from devices that shower a food with specific amounts of X-rays or beta rays. The Food and Drug Administraton (FDA) has approved doses of .1 Mrad or less (Mrad = Megarad or one million rads, the unit of measurement for radiation dosage). A review of forty years of use and experimentation with irradiated food products has led the World Health Organization, the Institute of Food Technologists and the American Medical Association to state that foods processed by irradiation are safe for consumption.

Of what benefit is this processing technique? Yearly, 25 to 30 percent of all fresh produce spoils through natural deterioration. Irradiation would extend this shelf life considerably. Food poisoning causes a great deal of illness and even a small number of deaths yearly. Irradiation could destroy the harmful bacteria. Currently the dose level approved by the FDA (.1 Mrad) is too low to accomplish this, but with expansion of irradiation and higher doses approved, salmonella food poisoning, affecting 2.5 million Americans a year, could be significantly reduced. The use of fumigants and insecticides could also be reduced as irradiation controls insect infestation.

Currently in the United States there is limited approval for the use of irradiation of food products. The four approved uses are:

1. Sprout inhibition of white potatoes (approved in the 1960s but not extensively used)
2. Insect disinfestation of wheat and wheat flour (approved in the 1960s but not extensively used; currently renewed interest since the fumigant EDB was banned in 1984)
3. Control of microorganisms and insects in spices and seasonings (approved in 1983 and used commercially)
4. Elimination of trichinosis in fresh pork (approved in 1985; limited use to begin in 1986)

Nutritionally the quality of irradiated food is good. Even at higher dose levels, not approved in the United States, nutrient losses are similar to those in canned foods. At low dose levels, nutrient loss is minimal; vitamin B_1 (thiamin) is the nutrient most affected.

Worldwide access to information on irradiation is currently available at the National Agricultural Library, Food Irradiation Information Center, Room 304, Beltsville, Maryland 20705.

-ITIS is a suffix meaning inflammation of a part of the body.

IU, or international unit, is a measure of biological activity. It is the amount of a nutrient that will cure deficiency symptoms in a laboratory animal. It is a different amount for different vitamins—for example, one IU of vitamin A does not weigh the same as one IU of vitamin D.

J

JIGGER refers to one and one half ounces, or 45 ml, of a liquid, usually alcohol. When preparing mixed drinks like gin and tonic, usually a jigger of gin is mixed with the tonic.

JOULE is an international unit for measuring heat or energy. It is expected that in the future food energy commonly measured in Calories will be given in joules. One Calorie equals 4.184 joules. To change Calories to joules, multiply by 4.2. An 80 Calorie apple would be 336 Joules.

JUNK FOOD, see Empty calorie food

K

KEFIR is a fermented milk originally used in the Caucasus Mountains of southeastern Europe. The fermentation process produces lactic acid and alcohol (about 1 percent). This tangy product is becoming more readily available in U.S. markets.

KETOSIS refers to the abnormally high accumulation of acidlike substances (ketones) in the blood, which disturbs the body's neutrality (pH balance), and can be dangerous. This condition is caused by too few available carbohydrates for normal metabolism of the ketones formed when fat is broken down. This may be due to uncontrolled diabetes, starvation or very low carbohydrate diets.

KIDNEY STONES form when salts precipitate out of the urine. They are made up of uric acid, cystine or more usually calcium. Calcium crystallizes with oxylates, phosphate and other substances. Many are passed spontaneously but others must be removed surgically. It is common practice to increase water consumption to reduce stone formation but it is not known whether or not this is effective. Calcium is usually not restricted unless intake is excessive. Thiazide diuretics (hydrodiuril) increase calcium reabsorption and lower the amount in urine so they may help reduce stone formation. High doses of vitamin C (4 gm or more a day) or a deficiency of vitamin B_6 (pyridoxine) increase oxalate excretion and the tendency to form calcium oxalate stones. Low purine diets have been used in the past to reduce uric acid stone formation but medication is the preferred treatment now.

See Purines

KILOCALORIES is a measurement used for food energy which is equal to 1000 calories (c). In this book the general term Calories (C) is used synonymously for kilocalories.

See Calories

KOSHER is a Hebrew word which means "permitted" according to the Torah, literally the law or the whole body of Jewish literature. Kosher, what is fit and proper to eat, is explained in the Jewish Dietary Laws, known collectively as *Kashruth*. Holiness is the fundamental reason for the Jewish Dietary Laws; hygienic value is incidental.

The separation of milk and meat is necessary; therefore, the two may not be prepared, cooked or eaten together. This separation leads to a classification of foods: "milchig" (milk and dairy products); "fleishig" (meat, fowl and products made from them); and "pareve," or neutral foods—fruits, vegetables, grains, fish, eggs—that can be eaten either with milk or meat.

Under each group there are foods that are unacceptable and cannot be eaten. Milk products that use meat or animal derivatives, like rennin, in their preparation are not allowed. Some additives, like glycerine, are not considered kosher. Kosher animals are those that both chew their cud and have a split hoof. This includes cattle, sheep, goats and deer. Animals that are not kosher are horses, donkeys, camels and pigs. Domestic fowl is kosher but wild birds and birds of prey are not. All meat and fowl must additionally be killed by a trained person called a *schochet*. The only pareve foods not allowed to be eaten are shellfish. All acceptable fish must have scales and fins. No convenience food is considered kosher unless it is certified by a rabbinical authority whose name or insignia appears on the package.

The Jewish homemaker may "keep kosher" to varying degrees of strictness. She arranges her kitchen to allow for the separation of meat and milk. She must have two sets of pots, pans, kitchen utensils, dishes, silverware, dishtowels and table linens; one set for dairy and one set for meat. Pareve foods can be prepared or eaten on either set. These kitchen items are stored, used and washed separately. Although it may appear to be a complicated process to maintain a kosher home, in practice this manner of food preparation and eating are a way of life and pose no problems for the homemaker.

KUMISS is a mildly acid milk product with relatively little alcohol (0.5 to 1.5 percent), native to Southern Russia. It is made from the milk of mares.

KWASHIORKOR is a severe protein deficiency disease. It is most common in underdeveloped areas of the world where it occurs when a child is weaned from the mother's breast milk and fed a low-protein cereal substitute. This often happens at a time when the need for protein is high and the food substituted does not contain enough protein. A bloated belly (edema), diarrhea, pigment changes in skin and hair, anemia and retarded growth are some symptoms. Risk of infection is great.

It can be prevented by feeding diets high enough in protein to meet the need of the weaned child. Treatment consists of a high-protein diet with enough calories.

L

LACT-AID is an enzyme preparation that acts on the
sugar in milk (lactose) and changes it to a more digestible form. Available in drug stores, it is useful for people with lactose intolerance which is caused by insufficient production of the enzyme lactase. A few drops of
Lact-Aid is added to a container of milk the night
before it is to be used. By morning the milk will contain
little lactose and so can be drunk comfortably by lac-
tase-deficient people.

In some areas, milk, ice cream and cheese treated
with Lact-Aid is available.

See Lactose, Lactose intolerance

LACTOSE, or milk sugar, is a dissacharide found in
milk, both skim and regular. Lactose is also used in
nutritional supplements, as a filler in the sugar substitute Equal, and in some other medications.

See Lactose intolerance

LACTOSE INTOLERANCE is an inability to digest
milk sugar, lactose, due to decreased amounts of the
intestinal enzyme *lactase*. People with this disorder

develop gas, diarrhea, cramps and bloating after they drink milk or eat food containing milk. The undigested lactose stays in the intestine, drawing in water like a laxative and fermenting to produce gas.

As infants most people have normal lactase activity but levels of lactase in some people decrease with age. In others low lactase levels occur because of intestinal infection, pregnancy or other conditions. Africans, Greeks and Orientals are more likely to suffer from lactose intolerance than are people of north European ancestry, but many adults of all ethnic groups have it.

Some people with lactose intolerance can use small amounts of milk without bad effects. If milk is taken with meals, it is easier to tolerate. Chocolate milk is less likely to cause a reaction. Hard cheese, yogurt and cultured buttermilk usually contain little of the lactose in milk so they are good substitutes.

See Lact-Aid, Lactose

LAETRILE is a cyanide-containing compound, also known as amygdalin, which has been added to herbal medicines for thousands of years. In 1920, Ernest Krebs rediscovered amygdalin, claiming it had anti-cancer properties. But so many of the patients he treated had toxic reactions that he abandoned his work. In 1952, Ernest Krebs, Jr., registered amygdalin with the U.S. Patent Office under the trade name *Laetrile*.

Supporters of this controversial cancer treatment claim that Laetrile is toxic only to cancer cells. In actuality it can result in cyanide poisoning and death. When taken orally, Laetrile reacts with an enzyme found in the gut, forming hydrocyanic acid. This acid, a cyanide, attacks the respiratory system and can cause death in as little as thirty minutes. Smaller doses result in nerve and skin damage.

Research does not support the use of Laetrile to cure, stabilize or improve cancer. The Food and Drug Administration has banned its sale in the United States.

Laetrile is sometimes referred to as vitamin B_{17}, implying that it is one of the B vitamins. It is neither a vitamin nor an effective cancer treatment and its use can result in illness and death.

See Amygdalin, Cancer

LAXATIVES are foods or drugs that will counteract constipation by causing bowel movements. Bran and other high fiber foods draw water into the intestine and swell, softening the stool and speeding its passage. Bulk producers like Metamucil, Cologel and Hydrolase act in the same way as fiber. Colace, Diconate and Surfak are medications that soften the stool in the same way.

Lubricants, like mineral oil, grease the lining of the intestine and also soften the stool. Habitual use of mineral oil can cause a vitamin loss because the fat soluble vitamins—A,D,E,K—dissolve in it and are carried out of the body.

Saline laxatives like Epsom Salts, Milk of Magnesia, Sal Hepatica and Fleet Phospho-Soda hold and draw water into the intestines. Thus, water is lost along with some minerals; both need to be replaced.

Irritant laxatives like Dulcolax, magnesium citrate, Feen-a Mint, Senokot and Cascara Sagrada stimulate intestinal movement. They often cause cramping.

All laxatives should be used for only short periods. Extended use can cause dependency and also loss of water, minerals and vitamins.

See Mineral oil

LDL is an abbreviation for low density lipoproteins.

See Lipoproteins

LEAD is a mineral that has toxic effects in the body causing anemia, kidney and nervous system damage. The lead in our bodies comes from water pipes, pesticides, automobile emission, paint and cans. Lead is used to seal or solder "tin" cans containing evaporated milk, tuna, fruit juice, etc. Canners have reduced the amount of lead used in cans, reducing the lead intake from this source. All lead solder has been removed from the construction of cans used for infant formula.

See Hair analysis

LECITHIN is a fatty substance containing choline that is used as a food additive in baked goods, margarines, salad dressings, ice cream and chocolates. It acts as an emulsifier, keeping fat dispersed in the product. In the body, lecithin prevents abnormal accumulation of fat in the liver.

Lecithin has been suggested as effective in treating high cholesterol levels in the blood. Some animal experiments in which lecithin was injected subcutaneously (beneath the skin) seem to support this. However, the effect of taking lecithin by mouth, as a supplement, has not yet been determined.

Lecithin and its component choline are being studied as a treatment for memory disorders. Lecithin, when used in clinical situations such as this, refers to a specific substance—Phosphatidyl-choline, a choline-containing substance. When the term lecithin is used in the food industry it refers to a whole family of substances (phosphatides) and may not contain much choline. This is true of lecithin granules used as a dietary supplement.

See Acetylcholine, Choline, Neurotransmitters

LIFE SPAN, the number of years that a person lives, has increased over the years because of improved medical care and social environment. A Roman baby born 2,000 years ago had a life expectancy of only 22 years. In 1900, average life expectancy was 49 years; in 1949, 68 years.

A baby born in 1984 can be expected to live, on the average, 74.7 years. White women have the greatest life expectancy—84 years. The life expectancy for black women is 80 years; for white men, 72 years; and for black men, 67 years.

Although the average life span is increasing, the maximum life span has increased very little. It is believed that man has a real upper limit of about 115 years and that even if killer diseases of later life like heart disease and cancer were reduced, probably no more than ten years would be added to average life.

LINOLEIC ACID is an essential fatty acid, a fat that cannot be made by the body and must be obtained from food. Deficiency has occurred in infants fed nonfat milk for long periods. A deficiency is not likely in adults because they have large fat stores in their body. Rich food sources are safflower oil, sunflower oil, corn oil, cottonseed oil, soybean oil, margarines made with these oils, and walnuts.

The average American diet provides 5 to 10 percent of its calories as linoleic acid. This more than meets the estimated requirement—3 to 4 percent of total calories for infants; 1 to 2 percent of total calories for adults.

See Fat

LIPOPROTEINS are packages of fat wrapped in water soluble protein. These combinations of protein, cholesterol and other fats carry cholesterol around in the blood. Cholesterol, because it is a fat, cannot dissolve in the blood which is mainly water.

The two most important kinds of lipoproteins are low density lipoproteins (LDL) that carry 50 to 75 percent of all blood cholesterol and high density lipoproteins (HDL) that carry 15 to 25 percent.

The LDL cholesterol is believed to be deposited into the coronary arteries, so when LDL's are elevated there is a greater risk of atherosclerosis. HDL cholesterol is carried to the liver which breaks it down and excretes it. Therefore a higher level of HDL is desirable as it indicates less risk of coronary artery disease. Normal range for HDL is 30 to 80 mg/dl. A value below 30 may indicate risk while values over 75 indicate a protective factor or decreased risk. HDL levels are high in premenopausal women, thin people, non-smokers, those who exercise regularly and who drink alcohol moderately (one to two drinks daily).

See Cholesterol, Heart attack

LIQUID OR FLUID DIETS are used when a person cannot tolerate solid foods. They may be either clear fluid or full fluid. The clear fluid diet is usually used for one or two days when food cannot be eaten; as the condition improves, i.e. surgery, dental work, a virus, a full fluid diet can be used.

Clear fluids: Water, chopped ice, tea with sugar, coffee, fat-free broth, flat soda (carbonated drink), strained fruit juice, synthetic fruit juice, fruit ice and plain gelatin.

Full fluids: All clear fluids plus milk, strained soups, cereal gruels, fruit and vegetable juices, custard, plain ice cream, sherbet and plain pudding.

The clear fluid diet supplies very few nutrients; it merely replaces fluids lost. The full fluid diet can be used for longer periods.

LITE OR LIGHT FOODS contain less of something like salt (sodium), fat, sugar or alcohol and are usually lower in calories. "Lite" beer is lower in alcohol and calories. "Lite" potato chips contain less sodium and fat and are lower in calories. When the term light is used to represent a claim for weight control, the foods must conform with the regulations for low- and reduced-calorie foods.

See Low calorie foods

LITE SALT, *see* Salt substitutes

LOW BIRTH WEIGHT is a term used to label a birth weight of 5½ pounds (2,500 grams) or less. It is often a predictor of poor health in the newborn and an indicator of probable poor nutrition by the mother during pregnancy. Normal birth weight is 6½ pounds (3,500 grams) or more.

LOW-CALORIE DIET, *see* Diet

LOW-CALORIE FOODS can only make this claim on the label if they contain no more than 40 Calories per serving. Foods that are naturally low in calories, like celery, may claim on a label to be "low-calorie."

Another category of low calorie foods are *reduced-calorie foods*. These foods must have at least one-third fewer calories than an equal serving of the food they are substituting for. The label of reduced-calorie foods must clearly list the calorie content of a serving along with the calorie content of a serving of the food it is replacing. The reduced-calorie substitute must be similar in taste, smell and "mouth feel" and not be nutritionally inferior.

LOW-CARBOHYDRATE DIET, *see* Diet

LOW-CHOLESTEROL DIET is used when a person has elevated serum cholesterol levels or simply as a prudent diet change to reduce the risk of heart attack.

A diet planned to lower cholesterol levels is generally low in calories (to help weight loss), contains no more than 30 percent fat (20 percent as unsaturated fat) and no more than 300 mg of cholesterol daily.

Liquid vegetable oils—corn, soybean, sunflower, safflower, cottonseed, olive oil—should be used instead of solid fats. Choose margarines with liquid vegetable oil as the first ingredient.

Beef, veal, lamb, pork and ham should be eaten in small portions, no more than three times a week. Use fish, chicken and turkey and twice a week substitute dried peas, beans or lentils for meat. Use lean meat trimmed of all fat and cook it without added fat. Avoid liver and other organ meats.

Skim milk and skim milk cheese should be used and eggs limited mainly to use in cooked foods. Coffee whiteners and nondairy whipped toppings should be avoided. Increase fiber from vegetables, fruits and whole grain cereals.

See Cholesterol, Low-fat diet

LOWER ESOPHAGEAL SPHINCTER (LES) is the muscle around the opening between the esophagus (food tube) and the stomach.

See Heartburn, Hiatus hernia

LOW-FAT DIET is a food plan that cuts down the percentage of calories coming from fat to 30 percent or less. This can be compared with the usual intake in the U.S. of about 43 percent of calories.

See Low-cholesterol diet

Eating Tips for a Low-Fat Diet

- Use liquid vegetable oils. Corn, soybean, sunflower, safflower, cottonseed (labeled Vegetable Oil), peanut and olive oils.

- Choose margarines with "liquid vegetable oil" as their first ingredient. When margarines are high in polyunsaturated fat, they give this information on their label.
- Limit beef, lamb, pork or ham. These foods should be eaten (in small amounts, 3–4 oz) only three times weekly. Use more fish, chicken, turkey and veal. Shellfish can be substituted for meat. Do not use liver or other organ meats. Use dried peas and beans and lentils in place of meat two or more times weekly.
- Use lean cuts of meat. Trim off all visible fat. Cook without added fat. Bake, broil or roast to further reduce fat.
- Use skim milk and skim milk cheese and yogurt. No butter, cream, sour cream or whole milk should be used.
- Avoid nondairy creamers and whipped toppings. Coffee whiteners and nondairy whipped toppings are high in saturated fat.
- Use fruits and vegetables. Use all types raw or cooked, without added butter, cream or sauce. Avoid avocado, olives and coconut.
- Limit eggs. Eggs should be limited to three a week, cooked without butter. Egg whites can be used as desired: 2 egg whites = 1 egg.
- Use cereals, rice, macaroni. Whole-grain varieties offer fiber and nutrients. Avoid granola cereals and sauces made with fat.
- Use sparingly nuts, seeds, chocolate, peanuts and peanut butter, all of which are high in fat.

Copyright: A. B. Natow and J. Heslin, *Nutritional Care of the Older Adult,* Macmillan, 1986.

LOW-FAT FOODS do not at this time have a regulated meaning. The Food and Drug Administration, however, has approved the following definitions that may be adopted into regulation in the future.

LOW FAT: A food containing less than 10 percent fat on a dry weight basis and not more than 2 grams fat per serving.

REDUCED FAT: A food with a fat content reduced by at least 50 percent as compared to the food it replaces.

See Lite or light foods, Low-calorie foods

LOW SALT DIET, *see* Low-sodium diets

LOW-SODIUM DIETS are eating plans that reduce the sodium (salt) content in food eaten. They are used to treat high blood pressure, edema (accumulation of fluid), kidney disease and heart failure. Sodium is part of table salt which is 40 percent sodium and 60 percent chloride. There are different levels of sodium restriction. A moderate sodium-restricted diet will allow an intake of about 2 to 4 grams of sodium a day. That is the amount in 5 to 9 grams of salt, about 2 teaspoons. This level of intake is sometimes called the "no-salt-shaker diet" because although small amounts of salt can be used in cooking, no additional salt is added at the table. Foods that must be avoided or used in very limited amounts include all salted and smoked meats and fish (bacon, ham, bologna and other luncheon meats, anchovies, salt cod), and condiments (seasoned salt, garlic salt, bouillon cubes, catsup, regular soy sauce and Worcestershire sauce). Salted chips, nuts, popcorn, pickles, olives and pretzels should also not be eaten.

Some usually salty foods like cheese and peanut butter now can be bought in low-salt versions.

Food additives with the word "sodium"—for example, sodium nitrite and sodium benzoate—can add more sodium to intake as can use of sodium containing antacids like Alka-Seltzer and Sal Hepatica.

Sometimes a more severely sodium-restricted diet is needed. In that situation, high-sodium vegetables like beets, carrots, kale, white turnips, dandelion greens, mustard and beet greens, spinach and Swiss chard are limited. Regular canned vegetables, vegetable juices, soups, meat and fish may not be used. Commercially baked breads and cakes—unless labeled "low-sodium"—should not be eaten. Meat, milk, and milk products are permitted in limited amounts.

See Salt, Salt substitutes, Sodium

M

MACROBIOTIC FOODS, *see* Zen macrobiotics

MAGNESIUM is an essential mineral. The 20 to 30 grams found in the body are mainly in the bones with lesser amounts in other tissues—blood, liver, muscles. About 30 to 50 percent of the magnesium in food is absorbed. Protein, lactose (milk sugar), vitamin D, growth hormone and antibiotics increase absorption. Absorption is decreased by high intake of calcium, unabsorbed fat, oxylates from spinach and chocolate, and phytates from grains. Drinking alcohol and taking diuretics (water pills) increase magnesium losses in urine.

Magnesium is part of bones and teeth and part of enzymes involved in metabolism. It has a relaxing effect on nerves and muscles. A deficiency of magnesium seen in cases of alcoholism, cirrhosis of liver and severe vomiting can cause muscle tremors, confusion, and loss of appetite.

The RDA for magnesium is 350 mg a day for adult men and 300 mg a day for adult women. Larger amounts are needed in pregnancy and breast feeding. The allowance for children ranges from 50 mg in infancy to up to 400 mg for adolescent males. Good food sources are dairy products, breads and cereals, green leafy vegetables, dry peas and beans and nuts.

Magnesium is part of the green color pigment in vegetables (chlorophyll).

See Minerals

MALNUTRITION refers to poor health resulting from a lack, imbalance or excess of the nutrients needed by the body. Classic nutritional deficiency diseases like scurvy and beri-beri are hardly ever seen in the United States. The rare exceptions are usually found in alcoholics or in neglected children. Nutrient excesses or imbalances are more often found. Obesity is almost universal as is dental decay and osteoporosis. These are due, in part at least, to excesses and imbalances.

See Undernourished

MANGANESE is an essential mineral found in the body in small amounts—12 to 20 mg. Manganese is involved in bone formation and growth of connective tissues and is an activator of many enzymes that function in metabolism. The role of manganese may be interchangeable with copper, zinc and iron in some instances. About 45 percent of the manganese in food is absorbed.

The safe and adequate range of manganese intake for adults is 2.5 to 5.0 mg a day. Recommendations for children range from 0.5 to 3.0 mg a day. Good food sources are dried peas and beans, nuts and wholegrain breads and cereals.

See Minerals

MANGO is a tropical fruit that can be eaten ripe or made into a juice or preserve. Unripe mangoes are made into pickles or chutneys. Worldwide, the mango ranks seventh among the top twenty most-eaten fruits in the world. One medium mango has 65 Calories, 11,000 IU of vitamin A (an unusually rich source— more than twice our daily need) and 70 mg of vitamin C, slightly more than is recommended daily.

MANNITOL is a sugar alcohol. It is 70 percent as sweet as sugar with one-half the calories. It is used in candies, baked products and chewing gum. Mannitol is used as a sweetener in some diabetic foods. Excess mannitol (10 to 20 gm) can cause diarrhea.

See Sorbitol

MARGARINE is a nondairy butter substitute. It contains the same amount of fat (80 percent) and calories (35 per teaspoon) as butter. The difference is that the fat in margarine usually is vegetable fat not animal fat. Because of this, there is no cholesterol in margarine and less saturated fat. At the same time margarine has larger amounts of the more preferable oleic acid (monounsaturated) and of linoleic acid, an essential fatty acid.

See Fat

MARIJUANA is a hallucinogenic plant, dried and smoked as a cigarette. The active ingredients are rapidly and completely absorbed from the lungs, transported by proteins in the blood to fat where it is stored. Marijuana remains in the body fat and is excreted slowly taking from several days to a week or more for the body to rid itself of the stored residue after smoking a single marijuana cigarette.

Marijuana has characteristic effects on hearing,

touch, taste, smell, and on the perception of time, space and the body. It can also produce alterations in sleep. Among the taste changes induced is a greater enjoyment in eating, especially of sweet foods. The mechanism of this effect is unknown since the drug does not alter blood sugar levels and prolonged use does not bring about a weight gain. Marijuana also alters heart action, often causing a rapid or irregular heartbeat. It reduces the body's immune response and reduces the level of sex hormones and sperm count in men. It is excreted in significant amounts in the milk of a nursing mother. Because it is banned for sale in the United States, there is no regulation of quality. Samples have been found to be contaminated with pesticides, heavy metals, as well as other "hard" drugs.

MAX-EPA, *see* EPA

MEASUREMENT SYSTEMS, metric and English, are used throughout the world for specifying length, area, volume and weight. Each system has its own unit of measure with specific relationships between the units. The English system has evolved through customary usage over many years with various uneven relationships between units. The metric system is more precise, based on multiples of ten (the decimal system).

LENGTH:

Metric:	millimeter	(mm) =	$1/1000$ of a meter (0.001)
	centimeter	(cm) =	$1/100$ of a meter (0.01)
	decimeter	(dm) =	$1/10$ of a meter (0.1)
	kilometer	(km) =	1000 meters

English:	12 inches	(in) =	1 foot (ft)
	3 feet	(ft) =	1 yard (yd)

WEIGHT:
Metric: The gram is the standard unit of weight. All weight units are based on the gram.

microgram (mcg) = $\frac{1}{1,000,000}$ gram (0.000001)
milligram (mg) = $\frac{1}{1000}$ gram (0.001)
centigram (cg) = $\frac{1}{100}$ gram (0.01)
decigram (dg) = $\frac{1}{10}$ gram (0.1)
kilogram (kg) = 1000 grams

English: 16 ounces (oz) = 1 pound (lb)
2,000 pounds (lbs) = 1 ton

VOLUME:
Metric: The liter or fraction of the liter are the standard unit of volume.

microliter (mcl) = $\frac{1}{1,000,000}$ liter (0.000001)
milliliter (ml) = $\frac{1}{1000}$ liter (0.001)
centiliter (cl) = $\frac{1}{100}$ liter (0.01)
deciliter (dl) = $\frac{1}{10}$ liter (0.1)
kiloliter (kl) = 1,000 liters

English: 8 ounces (oz) = 1 cup (c)
2 cups = 1 pint (pt)
2 pints = 1 quart (qt)
4 quarts = 1 gallon (gl)

Conversions between metric and English systems:
1 pound = 454 grams
1 inch = 2.54 centimeter
2.2 pounds = 1 kilogram
1 quart = 946 milliliters

MEGADOSES refers to taking large amounts of a substance. In the case of vitamins, ten or more times the RDA is considered a megadose. The RDA for vitamin C for adults is 60 mg; therefore, 600 mg or more of this vitamin would be a megadose. Megadoses can lead to hypervitaminosis and can cause negative side effects in the body.

See Hypervitaminosis

Risks From Taking Excess Vitamins

Vitamin	Symptoms of Overdose
Provitamin A (carotene)	Yellowing of skin
A	Loss of appetite; dry, itching skin; hair loss; joint swelling; enlarged liver
B_1 (thiamine)	None have been reported
B_2 (riboflavin)	Urine is bright yellow-orange color; no ill effects reported
Niacin	Acid form (nicotinic acid) causes flushing, burning and tingling around neck, face and hands; can cause high levels of uric acid and sugar in blood; liver damage
B_6 (pyridoxine)	Loss of muscle coordination; abnormal functioning of nervous system; numbness in hands and feet
B_{12} (cyanocobalamin)	None have been reported
Folic acid	None have been reported;* can mask symptoms of pernicious anemia
Pantothenic acid	None have been reported
Biotin	Can decrease normal production of stomach acid
C (ascorbic acid)	Diarrhea; addiction with possibility of rebound scurvy; increased absorption of iron; increased excretion of uric acid; increased risk for gout and uric acid kidney stones; interferes with urine test for sugar in diabetics; can mask presence of

Vitamin	Symptoms of Overdose
	blood in stool; decreased resistance to infections; damage to tooth enamel; anemia; destruction of vitamin B_{12}
D	Loss of appetite; nausea; headache; vomiting; excess urination; diarrhea; fatigue; calcium deposits in kidneys and other organs; high blood pressure; damage to artery walls; elevated blood cholesterol
E	Nausea; headache; increased blood clotting time; increased blood pressure in persons with high blood pressure; fatigue; muscle weakness; blurred vision; reduced activity of thyroid gland
K	Bleeding; kidney damage; anemia

*Persons on Dilantin should not take more than RDA of folic acid.

METABOLISM is the sum of all the chemical reactions, both cellular and subcellular, that occur to nutrients in the body. Metabolism has two phases: catabolism and anabolism. Catabolism refers to liberating energy from protein, fat or carbohydrate for the body's immediate demands. Anabolism is the process during which nutrient molecules are used as the building blocks to synthesize new body tissue (cells, hair, skin). This process supports the body's growth and repair needs. All body reactions are set in motion by the action of enzymes which are molecules that speed up a body process without being used up during it or entering directly into the process. Vitamins, minerals and water cannot by themselves supply energy to the body but they are essential to the metabolic process, making up portions of enzymes or supplying an appropriate medium for the metabolic process to take place.

METHYLENE CHLORIDE is used in making some types of decaffeinated coffee. This chemical has been shown to cause cancer in laboratory animals. The residue of methylene chloride currently allowed in decaffeinated coffee is ten parts per million. The Food and Drug Administration considers that the risk from this level is extremely low, "no greater than one in one million and probably closer to one in 100 million." Coffee manufacturers claim they cannot produce a product with lower levels.

See Decaffeinated coffee

METHYLXANTHINES are a family of stimulants including caffeine, theobromine and theophylline. They act as stimulants to the heart muscle, central nervous system and stomach acid secretion. Methylxanthines are diuretics, causing increased urination; they also increase levels of sugar and free fatty acids in the blood.

Caffeine occurs naturally in coffee, tea, cocoa and kola nuts (cola). Theobromine is found in cocoa and theophylline in tea.

See Caffeine

MG/DL means milligrams per deciliter and is expressed as mg/dl. A deciliter equals 100 milliliters. This abbreviation is often used when measuring blood levels of various substances.

MICROWAVE OVENS cook by agitating the water

molecules in food, causing friction and heat. This method of cooking is up to 70 percent faster than usual methods. The food, however, will not brown in a microwave oven since the cooking temperature never exceeds boiling (212°F). Due to the lower cooking temperature and shorter cooking time, more B vitamins and vitamin C are retained. Food defrosted in a microwave also retains more nutrients. Defrosting on the kitchen counter can result in food poisoning as bacteria multiply rapidly on the defrosted outer layer while the center is still frozen. Defrosting overnight in the refrigerator, a safe procedure, requires planning ahead.

Microwaves are electromagnetic energy waves that are generated in the oven by a magnetron tube which converts electricity into electromagnetic radiation. The frequencies used for microwave cooking (915Mhz, 2450Mhz) are regulated by the Federal Communications Commission. Any substance which contains water, such as food, absorbs microwaves efficiently and grows hotter. Glass, paper, plastic and straw do not absorb the microwaves, so they make excellent cooking containers. They transmit the microwave energy to the food without being heated in the process. Metal causes the microwaves to be reflected off the surface which can result in a rebound, ricocheting effect that can damage the energy source of the appliance.

MIGRAINE HEADACHES, affecting between 10 and 20 million Americans, have been linked to food allergies. Some studies show that approximately 75 percent of migraine sufferers are allergic to five or more foods. When they are on diets restricting these "trigger" foods, their headaches become less frequent and severe and in some cases stop completely.

Some allergists believe that persons with migraine headaches are allergic to common foods like wheat, corn, milk and eggs. Other studies linked migraine headaches to tyramine-containing foods. Tyramine is an amino acid found in aged cheese, wine, chocolate and yogurt. As there may be a delayed response to these foods, it is not always easy to identify the connection. Children have been found to crave the foods that provoked the headaches.

Not all authorities accept the importance of food allergy as a factor in migraine headaches. Some feel that there is not enough evidence as yet to warrant putting migraine sufferers on rigid, hard-to-follow diets.

See Allergy, Tyramine

MILK People drink milk from goats, water buffalo, mares and reindeer. In the United States we commonly drink cow's milk. Milk has been called a "perfect food" but it contains low levels of vitamin C and iron. It is, however, a good source of protein, calcium and vitamins B_2 (riboflavin) and D.

Milk can be bought with varying amounts of fat:

whole milk = 3.5–3.7% fat	=	160 C/cup*
2% milk = 2% fat	=	120 C/cup
1% milk = 1% fat	=	100 C/cup
fortified skim milk = .6% fat	=	90 C/cup
skim milk = less than 1% fat =		80 C/cup

*Calories per cup

Almost all milk is pasteurized, or heated, to destroy most harmful bacteria. Homogenization breaks up the fat in the milk so it stays in tiny droplets throughout the milk. Milk is fortified with 400 international units (IU) of vitamin D per quart. Some skim milk is also fortified with 2000 IU of vitamin A per quart.

Nondairy creamers are not made with milk and are not nutritionally equal to milk.

MILLIEQUIVALENTS (mEq) refers to concentration of a substance per liter of solution calculated by dividing the concentration in mg percent by the molecular weight.

Sodium is sometimes measured in milliequivalents and other times as milligrams. To convert milliequivalents (mEq) to milligrams (mg) multiply the number of mEq of the sodium by 23.

$$20 \text{ mEq} \times 23 = 460 \text{ mg of sodium.}$$

MINERAL OIL is a mixture of liquid hydrocarbons made from petroleum. It is used as a lubricant to relieve constipation. It should not be taken close to mealtimes as it can reduce the absorption of fat-soluble vitamins—A,D,E,K—which dissolve in the mineral oil and are carried out of the body with the unabsorbed mineral oil.

See Laxatives

MINERALS are inorganic compounds (they never have been part of a living thing), smaller than vitamins, and found in simple forms in foods. There are twenty to thirty different minerals important in nutrition which are consumed daily by eating a wide variety of foods. Like vitamins, minerals are not a source of energy (Calories) in the body. Minerals retain their identity in the body and cannot be converted into another form. This indestructibility helps to protect minerals in food, requiring no special handling to preserve them. Long soaking or cooking can leach minerals from a food, but if the cooking water is used for gravies or eaten in another way the minerals are not lost.

Minerals have many important functions in the body. Some become part of the body, such as the calcium and phosporous found in bones and teeth and the iron found in red blood cells. Others float in body fluids, giving these fluids (blood, sweat, urine) certain characteristics. By virtue of being ionic (having a plus or minus charge) as well as water-soluble, minerals influence the acid-base balance of the body and help to keep water distributed correctly in the cells and in the fluids surrounding them.

Some minerals like iron, copper, chlorine, magnesium, manganese, iodine and fluorine are stored in the body and can be toxic when taken in excess amounts. Other minerals, like sodium, can be readily excreted by the body and are not as likely to pose a risk of toxicity.

Because the amounts of minerals found in and needed by the body vary so greatly, they are often subdivided into two major categories: major minerals or macrominerals and trace minerals or microminerals. The macrominerals are needed in larger amounts each day, approximately 0.1 gm or more. They make up 0.1 percent of the body's weight. Trace minerals are needed in smaller amounts daily and make up a very small fraction of total body weight.

See Individual minerals, Megadoses, Multivitamin/mineral supplements

Major Minerals

	Function	Food Sources
Calcium	Builds bones and teeth; helps blood clot; aids muscle and heart function and nerve response	Milk, yogurt, cheese, ice cream, deep-green leafy vegetables, canned salmon, and sardines eaten with bones, tofu

	Function	Food Sources
Phosphorus	Builds bones and teeth, aids in muscle function and nerve response; used in many reactions in body	Milk, cheese, meat, eggs, whole grain breads and cereals, nuts, dry peas and beans, soda, phosphate food additives
Magnesium	Builds bones and teeth; aids in nerve response and muscle function; used in many reactions in body	Whole grain breads and cereals, nuts, meat, milk, dry peas and beans
Sodium	Maintains normal body state; needed for nerves and muscle function	Table salt, milk, meat, eggs, baking powder, carrots, beets, celery, spinach, bouillon cubes
Potassium	Maintains normal body state; needed for nerve and muscle function	Fruits, vegetables, whole grain breads and cereals, dry peas and beans
Chlorine	Maintains normal body state; part of normal acid in stomach	Table salt
Sulfur	Helps rid body of toxins; part of body protein; used in many reactions in body	Meat, eggs, milk, cheese, nuts, dry peas and beans

Trace Minerals

	Function	Food Sources
Iron	Builds red blood cells; helps release energy	Liver, meat, eggs, whole and enriched bread and cereals, dark-green leafy vegetables, nuts, dry peas and beans
Copper	Builds red blood cells; used to build bones and maintain nerves	Liver, meat, seafood, whole grain breads and cereals, dry peas and beans, nuts, cocoa
Iodine	Part of thyroid hormone	Seafood, iodized salt
Manganese	Needed for use of protein, sugar and fats	Whole grain breads and cereals, soy beans, dry peas and beans, nuts, vegetables, fruits
Cobalt	Part of vitamin B_{12}; makes red blood cells	Meat, liver, milk, eggs, cheese
Zinc	Used in many cell activities; needed for wound healing and normal growth	Liver, meat, eggs, seafood, milk, whole grain breads and cereals

	Function	Food Sources
Molybdenum	Used in cell activities	Liver, milk, whole grain breads and cereals, leafy green vegetables, dry peas and beans
Fluoride	Builds strong teeth and bones	Tea, fluoridated water
Selenium	Helps to release energy, protects body substances	Seafood, meats, whole grain breads and cereal
Chromium	Helps body use carbohydrates	Meats, whole grain breads and cereals, yeast
Nickel	Used in cell activities	Whole grain breads and cereals, dry peas and beans, vegetables, fruits
Tin	Used in cell activities	Meats, whole grain breads and cereals, dry peas and beans, vegetables, fruits
Silicon	Forms bone and cartilage	Vegetables, fruit, whole grain cereals
Vanadium	Found in teeth	Whole grain cereal and breads, root vegetables, nuts, vegetable oils

MINERAL SUPPLEMENTS, *see* Multivitamin/mineral supplements

MINERAL WATER, *see* Bottled water

MODIFIED FAST, *see* Diet

MODIFIED FOOD STARCHES are starches that have been modified to yield some unique or useful property helpful in food processing. Some methods of modifying food starches are conversion, cross-linking, derivatives, and pregelatinization. All of these methods yield a *modified* food starch which has one or more useful characteristics such as reduced thickness, extended gel life, increased cooking rate, increased cold water swelling (which permits thickening without cooking) and lowered gelatinization temperature. These modified food starches are used in many convenience products like instant puddings, imitation jellies, whipped toppings, gravies, frozen creamed sauces and baby foods.

Recently there has been some concern about the use of modified food starch in baby food and one major manufacturer has removed it from its product line. While modification changes the physical properties of starch, it has a minimal effect on the way that the body uses it. Young infants, under 3 months of age, have a limited ability to break down starches but after this age digestion of starch, whether modified or unmodified, appears to function normally. The American Academy of Pediatrics has recommended delayed introduction of solid foods (between 4 to 6 months of age) and most commercial baby food products that contain modified food starch are intended for use with older infants. Therefore, it is doubtful that digestibility problems related to modified starch used in baby food are a problem as long as sensible feeding practices are followed. Neither the Food and Drug Administration nor the

American Academy of Pediatrics has recommended removal of modified food starch from commercial baby food at this time.

See Baby food

MO-ER, *see* Tree ear

MOLYBDENUM is an essential mineral found in the body in tiny amounts—9 mg. It functions as part of two enzyme systems. The recommended range of intake is 0.15 to 0.5 mg a day and that amount is easily met by the diet. Good food sources are whole grains, wheat germ, dried peas and beans, and organ meats. There have been reports of toxic effects of molybdenum causing goutlike symptoms. Supplements of molybdenum should not be taken.

See Minerals

MONOPHAGIA is the desire or habit of eating only one kind of food.

MONOUNSATURATED FATS are found in animal and vegetable fats. Good sources are peanut oil, chicken fat, avocadoes, olive oil and rapeseed oil.

See Fat, Heart disease, Polyunsaturated fats, Saturated fats

MSG, monosodium glutamate, is a flavor enhancer with a long history. In 1908, a Japanese researcher, Professor Ikeda of Tokyo University, isolated monosodium glutamate from the seaweed *Laminaria Japonica*. For thousands of years before this, natural products rich in glutamate, such as sea tangle (a type of seaweed) and soy sauces, had been used in the Orient for their flavor-enhancing properties. In the United States, 30 million pounds of MSG is used yearly in a variety of foods.

In 1950, a research study reported allergies from MSG. Other research showed glutamate could cause toxic reactions in the brains of young mice. This led to concern about the safety of MSG as a food additive. At about the same time Dr. Kwok, a scientist from the University of Tokyo, identified the Chinese Restaurant Syndrome (CRS) and pointed to MSG as the cause.

The symptoms of the Chinese Restaurant Syndrome—sensations of warmth and tingling, stiffness and/or weakness of the arms and legs, headache, light-headedness, heartburn and stomach ache—appear related to MSG. This type of food intolerance is classified as a food idiosyncrasy rather than a food allergy. This food sensitivity does not involve the immune system and can be controlled by avoiding MSG.

A number of issues need to be examined more carefully to clearly understand the role of MSG in allergies, toxic reactions and CRS. The chemicals in MSG are not foreign to the body yet the action of these chemicals in the body and MSG's ability to enhance flavor are not clearly understood.

The early report of an allergic response to MSG resulted from using MSG made from sugar beets in the study. Currently 90 percent of the commercial MSG (including Accent) is extracted from sugar cane molasses; only 10 percent is made from sugar beets.

All of the animal research that showed a toxic effect of MSG was caused by taking MSG by injection. Eating MSG caused few problems. Nevertheless, in 1969, MSG was voluntarily removed from and its use was discontinued in commercial baby food.

The major problem with the widespread use of MSG is the high amount of sodium it adds to the food. For example, a serving of a dry soup mix may contain as much as 735 mg of MSG, containing approximately 50 milligrams of sodium.

The words monosodium glutamate or the initials

MSG must appear on the label in the list of ingredients. MSG will most typically be found in soups, canned chicken, frozen entrees, packaged stuffing mixes, seasoning and sauce mixes, and Oriental food products.

MULTIVITAMIN / MINERAL SUPPLEMENTS

come in so many varieties that it is impossible to make a generalization about what and how much they may contain. Most supplements on the market today contain a variety of vitamins and/or minerals. Some may provide only a single nutrient like calcium or vitamin C. Since a specific nutrient deficiency in the United States is rare, there is a great deal of debate over whether or not daily nutrient supplements are needed by healthy people. Irregular eating patterns, escalating food costs, lack of time, and dieting can all be barriers to eating well. There are few research studies evaluating the effect of a daily nutrient supplement on generally healthy people. The few that have been done tend to show a slight beneficial effect. Therefore, taking a vitamin/mineral supplement with dose levels at or below the RDA is certainly not harmful and in some instances may be beneficial.

For regulatory purposes, most vitamin and mineral supplements are considered as food substances and are not stringently regulated. The only supplements with regulated maximum potency levels are those formulated for use by children under age 12 and those for use by pregnant and breast-feeding women. The only nutrients regulated are the B vitamin folic acid and vitamin K.

Vitamins and minerals used in supplements can come from natural sources (for example, calcium from ground oyster shells or vitamin C from rose hips) or the nutrient may be derived chemically (synthetically). Synthetic supplements are identical in every way to their natural counterparts. They are made in a laboratory using the exact molecular model of the natural substance. Some argue that synthetic supplements contain inactive ingredients (the nutrients are considered the active ingredients) like waxes, sugars and artificial colors. Many *natural* supplements do also, and the label declaration of inactive ingredients may not always be reliable. What generally separates synthetic from natural supplements is the cost—the natural is usually more expensive. The key is to remember that the body will make use of either and in fact cannot tell the difference between the two.

The best nutrient supplement to buy is the least expensive brand that is approved for interstate commerce (guaranteeing purity and safety). Generic or store brands are often good choices as are those made by nationally known pharmaceutical firms.

See Megadoses, Minerals, RDA, Vitamins

MUSHROOMS are a highly esteemed food with over 38,000 varieties. They were eaten by primitive people long before the dawn of agriculture. Picking wild mushrooms, however, often proved risky and history records that Roman emperors, a couple of European kings and even a pope died of mushroom poisoning. The infamous Lucretia Borgia is suspected of doing in a few of her victims with poisonous mushrooms. Even today, cases of mushroom poisoning are reported each year to the National Clearinghouse for Poison Control. Clearly it is not wise to attempt to harvest wild mushrooms as there is no foolproof method for the average layperson of detecting the poisonous from the nonpoisonous. In some cases, only a few bites of a toxic mushroom can be fatal.

Cultivated mushrooms are perfectly safe and can be purchased fresh, frozen, canned or pickled. In the United States 60,000,000 pounds are harvested yearly.

The mushroom, a fungus, grows most readily on living trees, dead wood or in soil rich in organic matter. Horse manure is a major ingredient in the soil prepared for growing commercially cultivated mushrooms. These are the most common varieties of mushrooms.

Common cultivated mushrooms are the best known, have the traditional mushroom shape, a pale white color and a mild flavor.

Oyster mushrooms have a cap the color and shape of an oyster shell; grown in Europe and Taiwan.

Straw (Padi) mushrooms were first grown in China by rice farmers who saw the wild variety growing out of the straw left covering the rice paddies after the harvest. With an irregular high peak cap, straw mushrooms are commonly available dried.

Shitake mushrooms, which are grown on hardwood logs, have been eaten for over 2,000 years in China and Japan; currently they are becoming increasingly popular in the United States and are grown in California.

Truffles, the most expensive of mushrooms, are in fact not a true mushroom but a related fungus that grows underground near the roots of oak trees. The best varieties are from the Perigord region of France and the Piedmont area of Italy where they are harvested with the assistance of truffle-smelling dogs or pigs. Frenchmen believe that truffles enhance virility since Napoleon fathered his only son after dining on truffles.

All varieties are low in calories (2 in a small mushroom), and a good source of phosphorus, iron and niacin (a B vitamin).

N

NAPHTHOQUINONE is a chemical name for vitamin K.

See Vitamin K

NATURAL FOOD COLORS are made from plant and animal sources. They are more expensive, less stable and less rigorously regulated than synthetic food colors. Natural food colors account for about 10 percent of the color additives found in food. When a natural food color such as beet powder is added to a food it must be listed on the food label as an "artificial color." Here is a list of approved naturally occurring color additives:

Natural Color Substance	Source
annatto	seed pods of *Bixa orellana*
beets, dry powder	beets
beta-carotene	fruits, vegetables
caramel	heated sugar
carmine (cochineal)	female insects
carrot oil	carrots
fruit juice	fruit
grape skin extract	grapes

Natural Color Substance	Source
paprika	plant Capsicum annum
riboflavin (vitamin B_2)	plant and animal sources
saffron	stigmas of Crocus sativus
tumeric and oleresin	rhizome of Curcuma longa
vegetable juice	vegetables

NEUROTRANSMITTERS There are about twenty different substances that transmit impulses between nerve cells. Three of these neurotransmitters— serotonin, acetylcholine and norepinephrine—depend on the nutrients eaten in the last meal. A meal high in carbohydrate would allow more serotonin to be made in the brain. Another neurotransmitter, norepinephrine, is made in the brain from tyrosine, a protein fraction. Acetylcholine is made from the choline found in egg yolks, wheat germ and dried beans.

See Serotonin, Tryptophan

NIACIN, also known as nicotinic acid and niacinamide, is a member of the B family of vitamins. This vitamin acts as a coenzyme, often along with other B vitamins, in the release of energy from fat, carbohydrate and protein.

Niacin is easily absorbed, little is stored and the excess is passed out in urine. Niacin can be made in the body from the amino acid *tryptophan* and we get about 60 percent of the niacin we use from this source. The RDA for niacin is expressed as niacin equivalents (NE). An NE is 1 mg of niacin or 60 mg of tryptophan (the amount that can be converted to 1 mg of niacin). The RDA is 18 NE for adult males, 13 NE for adult females (with higher recommendations during pregnancy and breast feeding). Recommendations for children range from 6 NE for infants to 19 NE for young men. Good food sources of niacin are meat, poultry, fish, yeast, coffee, peanuts; for tryptophan, milk, eggs, dried peas and beans, peanuts and meat.

Niacin in large doses, up to 4 gm daily, has been used to lower cholesterol and protect against heart attacks. Mental illness has also been treated with large doses of niacin. The value of this is controversial. Two to 3 gm of the acid form of niacin, called nicotinic acid, can cause blood vessel dilation with flushing and itching of the skin. It can also cause liver damage and elevated blood glucose levels.

See Megadoses, Vitamins

Sources of Niacin

Food	Amount	Milligrams
Tuna, canned	3½ ounces	24.0
Product 19, Kellogg's	1 cup	20.0
Liver, beef	3 ounces	14.0
Jack in the Box		
Jumbo Jack Hamburger	1	11.6
Chicken	3 ounces	7.8
Tofu (soybean curd)	2 ounces	7.8
Corn Flakes, Kellogg's	1 cup	7.0
Peanut butter	2 tablespoons	6.8
McDonald's Quarter		
Pounder	1	6.5
Hamburger	3 ounces	5.1
Sugar Frosted Flakes,		
Kellogg's	1 cup	5.0
Carnation Instant Breakfast	1 envelope	5.0
Cottage cheese	½ cup	4.0
Avocado	½ medium	4.0
Peanuts	2 tablespoons	4.0
Brewer's yeast	1 tablespoon	3.9
Egg	1 large	3.0
Mango	1 medium	3.0
Raisin bran	½ cup	2.9

Food	Amount	Milligrams
Peas, cooked	½ cup	2.8
Potato, baked	1 medium	2.7
40% Bran Flakes, General Foods	½ cup	2.1
Sunflower seeds	2 tablespoons	2.0
Brown rice, cooked	½ cup	2.0
Pizza	1 slice	1.6
Banana	1 large	1.4
Guava	1 medium	1.4
Frankfurter roll	1	1.3
Puffed wheat	1 cup	1.2
Buttermilk	8 ounces	1.1
Wheat germ	2 tablespoons	1.1
Rice, cooked	½ cup	1.0
Whole-wheat bread	1 slice	.8
White bread	1 slice	.8
Cantaloupe	¼ melon	.8
Navy beans, cooked	½ cup	.7
Prune juice	4 ounces	.5
Milk	8 ounces	.2

The RDA for niacin is: 18 mg for males
                                   13 mg for females

The U.S. RDA (labeling tool) for niacin is: 20 mg

NICOTINIC ACID and niacinamide are chemical names for the B vitamin niacin.

See Niacin

NIGHTSHADE VEGETABLES include white potatoes, tomatoes, eggplant, peppers and apples. There are testimonials claiming that excluding these foods from the diet will eliminate pain and inflammation of arthritis. There is as yet no scientific basis for this claim. One theory, still unproven, is that some arthritis sufferers may be allergic to these foods and the allergic reaction causes the arthritic symptoms.

NITROSAMINES are compounds formed when nitrites in vegetables (beets, spinach, lettuce, radishes), saliva and food additives combine with amines (nitrogen combining substances). Nitrosamines are found in water, tobacco smoke, cured meats, alcoholic drinks and they may also be formed in our bodies. Nitrosamines have been shown to be powerful carcinogens in animal studies.

If vitamin C, as in orange juice, is eaten along with nitrite-containing foods, nitrosamine formation is prevented.

See Cancer, Vitamin C

NUCLEIC ACIDS are compounds that are carriers and transmitters of genetic information. DNA and RNA are the two nucleic acids found in humans.

NURSING BOTTLE SYNDROME occurs when an infant or very young child has extensive dental decay because a bottle, filled with a sweetened drink, is sucked on for extended periods during the day and through the night. As a sleepy baby sucks from a bottle, the tongue extends slightly out of the mouth and covers the lower front teeth. The sweetened drink (even milk contains the milk sugar lactose) bathes the upper teeth and lower back teeth. As the baby falls asleep, active sucking and swallowing slows down as does the flow of saliva. The drink tends to pool or puddle in the mouth surrounding the teeth and setting up a perfect environment to erode the enamel and start the process of cavity formation. With time and exposure, dental decay can become rampant, resulting in extreme cases in lost or broken primary teeth. The syndrome has also been identified in children who suck a pacifier dipped in a sweetener such as honey and in infants whose mothers ascribe to a prolonged at-will breast feeding regimen. Nursing bottle cavities can be prevented by establishing appropriate eating habits and by not allowing the infant or young child to sleep with a bottle. A bottle filled with plain tap water is a compromise for the older infant or child that is unwilling to give up the nighttime bottle.

NUTRASWEET, *see* Aspartame

NUTRIENTS are substances found in food that are necessary for life and health. We need over forty different nutrients including fat, carbohydrates, protein, vitamins, minerals and water. It is possible to get all needed nutrients in the foods we eat when food is chosen wisely.

See Individual nutrient names

NUTRITIONIST is usually a person with training in food science as it relates to growth, maintenance and health. Most nutritionists work in clinics, consultancies, public health, research and teaching. Some are employed in medical communications as journalists, reporters and editors. As the need for nutrition education increases the role of this profession will grow accordingly. In most states, however, there is no legal definition of the term nutritionist; therefore even someone without adequate training can use this title. The consumer should ask for background information to be sure that the nutritionist has adequate credentials; a degree in nutrition and an R.D. registration would be appropriate.

See Dietitian

NUTRITION LABELING is governed by law. In 1973 the Food and Drug Administration revised food labeling regulations and they continue to be subject to constant revision. Nutrition labeling is voluntary except for 1) foods such as enriched breads or fortified milk that have nutrients added and 2) those that make nutritional claims, such as breakfast cereals which claim they provide 100 percent of certain nutrients.

All nutrition labels follow the same format. The upper portion of the label shows the serving size, number of servings per container, calories per serving and the amount of protein, carbohydrate and fat per serving. The lower portion of the label lists the percentage of the United States Recommended Daily Allowance (U.S. RDA) for protein and seven vitamins and minerals provided in one serving. These must always be listed. If the amount of a nutrient is very low, an asterisk replaces the percentage and relates to a footnote stating "Contains less than 2 percent of the U.S. RDA."

If information on amount of cholesterol or type of fat appears on the label, the total grams of fat, percent of calories provided by fat, and grams of both saturated and polyunsaturated fat must be given.

Calorie claims are subject to these guidelines.

1. *Low calorie* is food containing 40 Calories or less per serving.
2. *Reduced calorie* is food having a calorie reduction of at least one third of the regular item.
3. *"For calorie restricted diets"* can be used if basis for claim is clearly stated.
4. *Diabetic foods* must state that food may be useful in the diet "on advice of a physician."
5. Terms *"dietetic," "diet,"* and *"artificially sweetened,"* are reserved for low-calorie, reduced-calorie or for calorie-restricted—diet foods.

Sodium (salt) content on label regulations went into effect July, 1986.

See U.S. Recommended Daily Allowances (U.S. RDA)

FDA Sodium Labeling Regulation

Descriptive Terms	(Per Serving)
"Sodium free"	less than 5 mg
"Very low sodium"	35 mg or less
"Low sodium"	140 mg or less
"Reduced sodium"	75% or greater reduction in sodium content
"Unsalted," etc.	no salt added in processing

The FDA's labeling regulation for potassium is voluntary and follows the same descriptive terms ("Potassium free," etc.) and increments as sodium.

—————————— O ——————————

OBESITY is an excess accumulation of body fat. Most experts agree that a person is considered obese when they are 20 percent or more over ideal body weight. Thirty-four million American adults fit into this category. Extreme or morbid obesity has been defined as twice the desirable weight or 100 pounds (45 kg) over desirable weight. Being overweight is a health risk. The degree of risk is variable depending on the amount of overweight and other risk factors that contribute to well-being.

There are many causes of obesity—excess calories, decreased physical activity, and metabolic and endocrine abnormalities. Although obesity has been linked to many illnesses, its greatest negative effect may be the enormous psychological burden it puts on those who are overweight.

There is a strong correlation between obesity and hypertension, hypercholesterolemia, noninsulin dependent diabetes and the incidence of certain cancers. Obesity can shorten a person's potential life span. This risk is greatest for those under 50 and increases with the duration and degree of overweight.

See Height/weight tables

OREO COOKIES are two chocolate cookie wafers filled with vanilla icing made by Nabisco. They are the best-selling cookie in the United States; 6 billion were sold in 1982. One Oreo cookie = 50 Calories.

ORGANIC FOODS, *see* Health foods

ORTHOMOLECULAR MEDICINE advocates the use of megadoses of vitamins—especially niacin, vitamin B_6 and vitamin C—in the treatment of schizophrenia and other ailments, including mental retardation, senility, hyperactivity, depression and learning disabilities.

Advocates of this treatment hope that the vitamins will increase enzyme activity and this will improve the medical conditions. Most of the claims for the value of this treatment are based on anecdotal reports—not scientifically controlled studies. When the American Psychiatric Association reviewed the available data, they rejected the claims that orthomolecular treatment is useful in treating mental illness.

See Megadoses

OSTEOARTHRITIS, or degenerative joint disease, is the most common form of arthritis. It develops because of wear and tear on the joints, from overuse, stress or injury. You are more likely to develop osteoarthritis as you get older. Although it is a chronic disease, it is usually mild.

Many dietary "cures" have been suggested for osteoarthritis—oil, apple cider vinegar, green-lipped mussel extract, rutin (a bioflavinoid), blackstrap molasses, lecithin, alfalfa, yucca extract and eliminating nightshade vegetables (white potato, tomato, eggplant, pepper and apples). Experts believe that nothing you eat can cause arthritis inflammation and nothing can cure it. When you read testimonials to the relief obtained when nightshade vegetables are not eaten, it may be that some arthritic sufferers are allergic to these foods and the allergic reaction is what causes the joint pain and inflammation. Another factor is that arthritis pain may be worse at some times than others even when no treatment is used. That is why it is difficult to tell how much relief is gained from diet changes.

See Arthritis, Nightshade vegetables

OSTEOMALACIA, or adult rickets, is a softening of the bones caused by a lack of vitamin D or the minerals calcium and phosphorus. An imbalanced ratio of calcium to phosphorus can also be a factor. The bones soften, becoming deformed; there may be bone tenderness and pain as well. Overuse of aluminum hydroxide antacids (Maalox, Mylanta) can cause osteomalacia by blocking phosphorus absorption. Calcium is lost from the body as the kidneys try to balance the level of these minerals in the blood.

Treatment consists of vitamin D and calcium supplements. Osteomalacia can be prevented by exposing the skin to sunlight so that vitamin D can be produced. If this is not possible, 400 to 800 IU of vitamin D can be taken daily along with eating calcium-rich food plus a calcium supplement so that calcium intake is at least 1,000 mg a day.

See Calcium, Vitamin D

OSTEOPOROSIS, or adult bone loss, refers to loss of bone mass which occurs in aging. The bone composition is normal but it becomes progressively thinner. When one third or more of the bone is lost, the bones fracture easily and do not heal well. Bone loss starts in both men and women as early as age 30, but the loss is accelerated in women at menopause (whether surgical or natural menopause). One in four postmenopausal women develop osteoporosis, while in men over 65 only one in eight is affected. Women may be more susceptible because they start out with smaller bones, may be less active, often diet so they obtain an inadequate amount of calcium, may have multiple pregnancies and breast feed, which uses up the body's calcium reserves. Women also often live longer than men so they can be more easily affected by a progressive, chronic condition. Inadequate intake of calcium and vitamin D, excess protein foods, smoking, excess alcohol intake, regular use of antacids, thyroid supplements, fair skin, slender body and little exercise are other risk factors for developing osteoporosis. Loss of height, periodontal (gum) disease and inward curvature of the spine may be indications that osteoporosis is developing.

Recommendations for avoiding or postponing the development of osteoporosis include:

- Take regular exercise.
- Eat calcium-rich foods daily, with a calcium supplement if total food intake is lower than 1,000 mg (the amount in 1 quart of milk).
- Drink fluoridated water.
- Expose skin to sunshine and/or get adequate amounts of vitamin D from fortified milk, margarine, fish oils or other supplements.
- Don't eat excessive amounts of meat or other high protein foods.
- Don't drink large amounts of soda.
- Don't take excessive amounts of antacids.

See Calcium

PABA (para-aminobenzoic acid) is part of folic acid, a B vitamin. It is sometimes touted as a separate essential nutrient but its only role in human nutrition is as part of folic acid. PABA is useful as a sunscreen. You will see it listed among the ingredients of suntan lotion. The preparations which contain the most PABA are more effective. Taking PABA as a supplement, sold in 50 and 100 mg tablets, is useless as a sunscreen. It can be harmful as it may help disease-causing bacteria to grow faster and become more resistent to some treatments. Large amounts of PABA, 10 grams or more, can cause a toxic reaction.

PANTOTHENIC ACID is a member of the B vitamin family. It is needed to make enzymes that regulate body processes. Although pantothenic acid is essential and important in normal body function, little is known about the exact human requirement for this nutrient. It is found in a wide variety of foods so there is little danger that anyone would become deficient. Its very name comes from the Greek word *panthos* which means "everywhere." It is estimated that the average American diet provides twice the recommended need. Claims that supplements of pantothenic acid are helpful to prevent or restore color to grey hair or cure diseases are unfounded. Supplements in excess of 10 grams (10,000 milligrams) a day may cause diarrhea.

See Vitamins

Sources of Pantothenic Acid

Food	Amount	Milligrams
Product 19, Kellogg's	1 cup	10.0
Carnation Breakfast Bar	1	2.0
Salmon steak	4 ounces	1.9
Brewer's yeast	1 tablespoon	1.2
Avocado	½ medium	1.1
Broccoli	¾ cup	.9
Egg	1	.9
Milk, regular	8 ounces	.8
Potato, baked	1 large	.8
Liver	3 ounces	.7
Brussels sprouts	4 large	.6
Strawberries	1 cup	.5
Cashews	2 tablespoons	.4
Cantaloupe	¼ melon	.3
Dill pickle	1 large	.3
Oatmeal, uncooked	¼ cup	.3
Dates	5 medium	.3
Whole-wheat bread	1 slice	.2

The RDA for pantothenic acid is: 4–7 mg

The U.S. RDA (labeling tool) for pantothenic acid is: 10 mg

PERIODONTAL DISEASE is a form of dental disease that affects the tissue and bone that anchor the teeth to the jaw. Bacterial plaque allowed to multiply unchecked eventually breaks down the tissue and bone, resulting in lost teeth. The plaque causes the gums to swell and turn red, often bleeding when brushed, in contrast to the pink color of healthy gums. Appropriate dental care, daily flossing of teeth and an adequate diet including optimal fluoride, vitamin D and calcium are helpful in preventing periodontal disease. Many experts believe periodontal disease is a predictor of osteoporosis (adult bone loss) in other parts of the body.

See Dental health, Osteoporosis

PERRIER WATER is a naturally carbonated low-salt mineral water bottled in France. One liter (little more than a quart) of Perrier water contains the following minerals:

$$
\begin{aligned}
\text{calcium} &= 140.2 \text{ mg} \\
\text{magnesium} &= 3.5 \text{ mg} \\
\text{sodium} &= 14.0 \text{ mg} \\
\text{potassium} &= 1.0 \text{ mg}
\end{aligned}
$$

See Mineral water, Bottled water

pH is a numerical scale representing acidity or alkalinity of substances. A pH 7.0 to 14.0 represents alkalinity; below 7.0 represents acidity. The pH of a lime is 2.0; the pH of egg white is 8.0.

See Acid

PHOSPHORUS is an essential mineral found in every cell and all body fluids. Eighty to 90 percent of the approximately 650 mg in the body is found in bones and teeth. Its other functions are buffering substances to maintain neutrality, controlling release and storage of energy, regulating hormones, and forming a structural component of cell walls, enzymes and nucleic acids.

About 70 percent of the phosphorus in foods is absorbed. Except for young infants, the RDA for phosphorus is the same as for calcium, ranging from 240 mg for infants up to 6 months to 1,200 mg for boys and girls 11 to 14. A deficiency of this mineral is not likely as the average intake in the United States is over 1,500 mg.

Good food sources are milk and milk products, eggs, nuts, dried peas and beans, meat, poultry and fish. Phosphorus-containing food additives are estimated to add approximately 500 mg daily. Deficiencies have been reported to occur in infants fed cow's milk and in persons taking large amounts of antacids. Excess intakes of phosphorus when coupled with low intakes of calcium may be a factor in the development of osteoporosis.

See Minerals, Nucleic acids, Osteoporosis

PICA is an abnormal craving for nonfood items like clay, dirt, plaster, paint chips and ice. Iron deficiency may be the cause in some cases.

POLYDEXTROSE is a reduced-calorie bulking agent aproved by the Food and Drug Administration in 1981. Polydextrose is not a sweetener but a substance that can replace sugar or fat in frozen desserts, cakes and candies, reducing calories by as much as 50 percent. The substance is a polymer prepared from dextrose with small amounts of sorbitol (a sugar alcohol) and citric acid. It is soluble in water and yields only 1 Calorie per gram, whereas fat and sugar have 9 Calories and 4 Calories, respectively, per gram. This food additive should allow the development of a wide array of high quality, reduced-calorie foods.

POLYUNSATURATED FATS are found in vegetable fats made from corn, cottonseed, safflower, sunflower and soybean. Vegetable fats are mainly polyunsaturated fatty acids. A few exceptions are coconut oil, palm oil and cocoa butter (chocolate). Vegetable oils may be hydrogenated (hardened) which makes them more saturated—for example, when margarine is made from corn oil. Do not be misled into thinking that all vegetable oil listed on a label is polyunsaturated. Coconut oil, a highly saturated vegetable oil, is frequently used.

See Fat, Heart disease, Monounsaturated fats, Saturated fats

POSTUM is an instant, caffeine-free, hot beverage made from bran, wheat, molasses, maltodextrin and natural coffee flavor. When prepared, according to package directions with 1 teaspoon per cup of water, it contains 12 Calories from 3 gm of carbohydrate and nothing else. It may look like coffee, but the flavor is somewhat different.

POTASSIUM is an essential mineral with about 250 gm in the average adult's body. Ninety-seven percent of the mineral is found within the body cells. Potassium's role, along with sodium, is in maintaining acid-base and fluid balance and also in transporting nutrients in and out of cells. Potassium is needed for insulin secretion and enzyme reactions; it also acts to relax the heart muscle in opposition to calcium which stimulates the heart.

The recommended safe and adequate intake of potassium is between 1,875 and 5,625 mg a day for adults. Lower amounts are suggested for children. Potassium is found in many foods; the average intake is estimated to be 2,000 to 6,000 mg a day. Good food sources are meats, poultry, fish, bananas, potatoes, tomatoes, carrots, celery, oranges and grapefruit.

Potassium deficiency, or hypokalemia, is usually not due to a dietary lack but it can occur in severe malnutrition. Prolonged vomiting, diarrhea, fever, severe burns and some diuretics can cause deficiency. Hypokalemia can cause rapid, irregular heartbeats, muscle weakness, nausea, vomiting and diarrhea. Hyperkalemia, or potassium toxicity, results from kidney failure, severe dehydration, or an underactive adrenal gland. It causes slow, irregular heartbeats and muscle weakness.

Potassium supplements or potassium chloride, should be used under a doctor's supervision. Misuse of these supplements has caused deaths. Some salt substitutes are potassium chloride compounds and these should be used with caution under medical supervision.

See Minerals, Salt substitutes

PPA (Phenylpropanolamine) is a stimulant, used as a nasal decongestant, vasoconstricter and more recently as an appetite suppressant. Five billion doses of this drug were sold in 1980. It is an ingredient in over-the-counter diet pills like Dexatrim, Prolamine and Dietac. It seems to work by dulling the sense of taste and smell. Food doesn't taste as good so less is eaten.

Reported side effects are increased blood pressure and damage to blood vessels in the brain, leading to even more serious disorders of the nervous system—confusion, stroke, psychotic behavior. Low doses of PPA may be safe as a short-term weight-loss aid for healthy people. Products containing PPA should not be used by persons with high blood pressure, heart disease, diabetes or thyroid disease or by pregnant women, nursing mothers or children under eighteen.

PRE-CONCEPTION NUTRITION refers to the nutritional requirements of a woman who is interested in setting the stage for a healthy pregnancy. It comes as a shock to many people to learn that 15 to 25 percent of all pregnancies do not result in a live birth. Most of these pregnancies end in a miscarriage which occurs in the first month. Every congenital malformation occurs in the first trimester (three months) of pregnancy. Both these events may occur before the woman realizes that she is pregnant and may happen before her first doctor's visit. In fact, 21 percent of all American women do not receive any prenatal care in the first three months of pregnancy. Current recommendations for optimal care during pregnancy suggest fourteen visits over nine months. More and more obstetricians are advising sixteen visits, beginning before conception.

The advantage of pre-conception counseling is to assess risks before conception. The major nutritional risk is weight. Women who are significantly overweight or underweight when they conceive are at increased risk for complications during pregnancy and their babies are at greater risk after birth. Ten percent under or 35 percent over ideal weight is defined as "at risk." The ideal time to lose or gain is before pregnancy. A pregnant woman should never diet in an attempt to keep her weight down.

Poor or bizarre eating habits can decrease the infant's birth weight, decrease the Apgar score (a rating system that predicts an infant's survival in the first month of life), and increase the incidence of toxemia, neural tube defects (incomplete closure of the spinal cord) and produce later learning problems. Excessive use of alcohol, caffeine or high doses of vitamins can also lead to problems.

Nutrition counseling before conception can help the woman achieve ideal weight and store needed nutrients that protect her and her unborn child. This will help to reduce the risk of complications, low birth weight, prematurity and some birth defects.

See Pregnancy

PREGNANCY refers to the period of time from conception to the birth of a baby. A full-term pregnancy takes approximately forty weeks or nine months. Women who eat well before conception and during pregnancy greatly increase their chances of having a healthy baby.

During pregnancy nutrient needs increase to support the growth of the fetus and support the health of the mother. The following table shows this increase for the major nutrients.

NUTRIENT	NONPREGNANT REQUIREMENT	PREGNANCY ADDITION
Energy (Calories)	1,600 to 2,400	+300
Protein	44 gm	+30 gm
Vitamin A	4,000 IU	+1,000 IU
Vitamin D	5 mcg	+5 mcg
Vitamin E	8 mg	+2 mg
Vitamin C	60 mg	+20 mg
B Vitamins		
Folic acid	400 mcg	+400 mcg
Niacin	13 mcg	+2 mg
B_1	1.0 mg	+0.4 mg
B_2	1.2 mg	+0.3 mg
B_6	2 mg	+0.6 mg
B_{12}	3 mcg	+1 mcg
Calcium	800 mg	+400 mg
Phosphorus	800 mg	+400 mg
Iodine	150 mcg	+25 mcg
Iron	18 mg	*
Magnesium	300 mg	+150 mg
Zinc	15 mg	+5 mg

*30 to 60 mg of supplemental ferrous iron per day is recommended.
Source: Food and Nutrition Board, National Research Council, National Acadmy of Sciences, in the Recommended Dietary Allowances, 9th ed., 1980.

Ideally the pregnant woman should gain 24 to 27 pounds, most of it in the second and third trimesters. This may sound like a lot but it is needed for a healthy

Food Groups

Food Group	Servings Per Day		Food Sources
	Pre-conception	Pregnant	
Milk major source of calcium	2	3 to 4	Milk, yogurt, cheese, ice cream, pudding, custard, sardines, salmon with bones, green leafy vegetables, shrimp, tofu (soybean curd)
Meat major source of protein and iron	4 ounces	6 to 8 ounces	Meat, fish, poultry, eggs, cheese, dried peas and beans, peanut butter, nuts, seeds, tofu (soybean curd)
Fruit and Vegetable major source of vitamins, minerals and fiber	4 or more 1 high in vitamin C 1 high in vitamin A	4 or more 2 high in vitamin C 1 high in vitamin A	All fruits and vegetables including potatoes Vitamin C-rich sources: orange, grapefruit, tangerines, tomatoes, strawberries, cantaloupe, raw cabbage, bok choy, broccoli, cauliflower, papaya, mango

			Vitamin A-rich sources: carrots, sweet potatoes, winter squash, pumpkin, chicory, endive, escarole, romaine, collard greens, kale, Swiss chard, turnip greens, spinach, apricots, cantaloupe, bok choy, broccoli
		4 or more	
		4 or more	Bread, rolls, bagels, cereal, rice, pasta, noodles, tortilla, waffle, pancake
Bread and Cereal	major source of energy, B vitamins, minerals and fiber		

placenta, uterus, blood, breast growth and healthy baby. The nutrients needed to support this growth come from the foods eaten. The diet should not be high in sugar, fat or alcohol.

The following food groups can be used as a guide to selecting a healthy food plan during pregnancy.

See Low birth weight, Pre-conception nutrition

PREMENSTRUAL SYNDROME, or PMS, refers to a range of symptoms including water retention, headaches, tender breasts, increased appetite, clumsiness, irritability, depression and anxiety. Not all women have the same symptoms. This condition occurs regularly, usually seven to ten days before the menstrual period begins, in 20 to 60 percent of American women. The cause is unknown but a variety of treatments have been tried—vitamins, hormones, tranquilizers and diuretics. Specific diet recommendations include decreasing caffeine (a possible cause of breast tenderness), reducing salt and sweets (to decrease water retention), reducing alcohol and eating small, frequent high protein meals.

PRESERVATIVES prevent unappetizing changes in color, flavor and texture of food and block the harmful effects of microorganisms. Following is a list of common food additives that act as preservatives.

Additive	Used in	Function
Alpha-tocopherol	vegetable oil	antioxidant
Ascorbic acid	oily food	antioxidant
erythorbic acid	cereal	color stabilizer
sodium ascorbate	soft drinks	
sodium erythorbate	cured meat	

Additive	Used in	Function
BHA (butylated hydroxyanisole)	cereals chewing gum baking mixes snack chips instant potatoes	antioxidant
BHT (butylated hydroxytoluene)	same as above	antioxidant
Calcium propionate or sodium propionate	bread rolls pie cakes	prevents mold growth
Citric acid sodium citrate	ice cream sherbet fruit drinks candy soft drinks instant potatoes gelatin desserts jam	antioxidant acidifier flavoring agent chelating agent
Lactic acid	Spanish olive cheese frozen desserts soft drinks	acidifier flavoring agent
Lecithin	baked goods margarine salad dressing chocolate ice cream	emulsifier antioxidant
Propyl gallate	vegetable oil meat products potato snacks chicken soup base chewing gum	antioxidant

Additive	Used in	Function
Sodium hypophosphite	bacon frankfurters smoked meat ham	preservative
Sodium benzoate	fruit juice soft drinks pickles preserves	inhibits growth of microorganisms
Sodium nitrate	ham frankfurters luncheon meat corned beef	coloring agent flavoring agent
Sodium nitrite	smoked fish bacon	preservative
Sorbic acid potassium sorbate	cheese syrup jelly cakes wines dry fruit	prevents growth of mold and bacteria
Sulfur dioxide sodium bisulfite	sliced fruit wine grape juice dehydrated potatoes	prevents bacterial growth bleaching agent

PROCESSING AGENTS are a group of food additives that aid in the production of food by improving taste and texture. Following is a list of commonly used processing agents.

Additive	Used in	Function

Alginate
  propylene glycol
  alginate
	ice cream
	cheese
	candy
	yogurt
	soft drinks
	salad dressing
	beer
		thickening agent
		foam stabilizer

Calcium stearoyl
  lactylate
Sodium stearoyl
  lactylate
Sodium stearoyl
  fumarate
	bread dough
	cake filling
	artificial whipped
	  topping
		dough conditioner
		whipping agent

Carrageenan	ice cream jelly chocolate milk infant formula	thickening agent stabilizing agent
Casein sodium caseinate	sherbet ice cream candy soft drinks instant potatoes	whitening agent thickening agent
Dipotassium phos- phate	cold cereals	chelating agent

EDTA
  ethylenediamine
  tetraacetic acid
	salad dressing
	margarine
	sandwich spread
	mayonnaise
	processed fruits
	  and vegetables
	canned shellfish
	soft drinks
		chelating agent

Additive	Used in	Function
Gelatin	powdered dessert mixes yogurt ice cream cheese spread beverages	thickening agent gelling agent
Glycerin glycerol	marshmallows candy fudge baked goods	maintains water content
Gums guar locust bean arabic tragacanth acacia	beverages ice cream frozen pudding salad dressing dough cottage cheese candy drink mixes	thickening agents stabilizers
Modified food starch	soup gravy baby food	thickening agent
Monoglycerides Diglycerides	baked goods margarine candy peanut butter	emulsifier
Pectin	jelly jam soft cheese	stabilizer thickener
Phosphoric acid phosphates	baked goods cheese powdered foods cured meat soda pop	acidulant chelating agent buffer emulsifier discoloration

Additive	Used in	Function
	breakfast cereal	inhibitor
	dehydrated	
	potatoes	
Polydextrose	frozen desserts	bulking agent
	cakes	
	candies	
Polysorbate 60	baked goods	emulsifier
	frozen desserts	
	imitation dairy	
	products	
Sodium carboxy-methyl cellulose methyl cellulose carboxymethyl cellulose (CMC)	ice cream beer pie filling icing diet food candy	thickening agent stabilizing agent prevents sugar from crystal-lizing
Sodium silicoalumi-nate	salt baking powder sugar	antifoaming agent anticaking agent
Sorbitan mono-stearate	cakes candy frozen pudding icing	emulsifier

PROOF refers to the concentration of ethanol (ethyl alcohol) in a liquid. In the United States proof is twice the ethanol concentration. Gin or vodka that is labeled 80 proof contains 40 percent alcohol. Wine which is usually 10 to 14 percent alcohol would be 20 to 28 proof. Drugs may also contain alcohol—for example, Geritol, which has 12 percent alcohol, is 24 proof; NyQuil, which has 25 percent alcohol, is 50 proof.

PROSTAGLANDINS are hormonelike substances made from essential fatty acids. They are involved in many body functions like muscle contractions, blood pressure, blood clotting, transmission of nerve impulses. The highest concentration of prostaglandins have been found in human semen.

PROTEIN, made up of amino acids, is found in every cell of the body and all of the body substances except for urine and bile. We get the protein we need to build our bodies from foods. The RDA is 56 gm for men and 44 gm for women. If you drink milk, eat meat, fish, poultry or beans, eggs or some nuts along with bread and vegetables, you will easily eat more than enough protein. In fact, most Americans eat more than twice as much as they need!

When you eat protein from animal sources like meat, fish, poultry, eggs, milk, or cheese, you are getting a full complement of all the amino acids you need. Protein from vegetable foods like cereal, bread, potatotes, rice, or beans contains some, but not all, of the amino acids we need to build body protein. When you eat a combination of these vegetable foods, you increase the assortment of amino acids available.

The average American eats about 14 percent of his or her total Calories as protein. Each gram of protein equals 4 Calories.

See Amino acids, Protein complementation

PROTEIN COMPLEMENTATION refers to eating two or more protein sources at the same time to enhance the overall protein quality of the meal or dish. Protein in different foods differs in quality. Protein quality refers to how well the protein can be used by the body to build and repair body cells. The protein in meat, fish, poultry, eggs and dairy products is of excellent quality because all of the essential amino acids are present in almost equal amounts. The protein in plants foods—grains, seeds, nuts, dried peas and beans—is of lesser quality. All of the essential amino acids are present but not in equal amounts. One or more of the amino acids is limited or available in only very small amounts. This is refered to as the *limiting amino acid*—the one that will run out first when the body is making new protein. Once one of the essential amino acids is used up, all the remaining amino acids from that food are useless to the body for manufacturing new protein. The leftover amino acids will be used for energy.

To improve the quality of plant protein, two or more plant proteins can be eaten at the same meal—protein complementation. The sum of the combined proteins will allow the body to make better use of all the amino acids eaten. By piggybacking two or more plant proteins one can achieve an amino acid mixture similar to meat. Another way to complement proteins is to put a small amount of animal protein with a larger amount of vegetable protein. Besides meat, fish and poultry there are six other categories of protein-containing foods—grains, legumes (dried peas and beans), nuts, seeds, milk products and eggs. We complement proteins all the time without even realizing it. For the vegetarian, protein complementation is essential to ensure adequate protein quality in the diet.

	Complemented proteins
Macaroni and cheese	grain + dairy foods (milk and cheese)
Peanut butter on whole wheat bread	legume + grain
Buckwheat pancakes	grain + egg + dairy food
Cereal and milk	grain + dairy food
Rice au gratin	grain + dairy food
Rice and beans	grain + legumes

Alternate Protein Foods

To make these foods high-quality protein, equal to meat, combine any food from one column with any food from another column of the same meal.

Grains	Legumes	Dairy Foods	Eggs	Nuts	Seeds
Barley	Black beans	Cheese	Any style	Almonds	Pumpkin seeds
Brown rice	Blackeyed peas	cottage		Brazil nuts	Sesame seeds
Buckwheat (kasha)	Chickpeas	natural		Cashew nuts	Sesame butter
Bulgur	(garbanzos)	processed		Chestnuts	(tahini)
Cornmeal	Kidney beans	Dry milk products		Coconut	Squash seeds
Cracked wheat	Lentils	Milk		Hazel nuts	Sunflower seed
Millet	Lima beans	Yogurt		Pecans	
Noodles	Mung beans			Pine nuts	
Oatmeal	Mung bean sprouts			Pistachio nuts	
Pasta	Navy beans			Walnuts	
Rice	Pea beans				
Rye	Peanuts				
Wheat berries	Peanut butter				
Wheat germ	Peas				
Whole wheat	Pinto beans				
	Soybeans				
	Soybean sprouts				
	Soy flour				
	Soy protein				
	Soy milk				
	Split peas				
	Tofu (soybean curd)				

Copyright: A. Natow and J. Heslin, *Nutrition For the Prime of Your Life*, McGraw-Hill, 1983

	Complemented proteins
Minestrone soup	grain (pasta) + legumes
Yogurt with wheat germ	dairy food + grain +
and walnuts	nuts
Sesame seed roll	seed + grain

See Protein, Vegetarianism

PURINES are nitrogen-containing compounds that are not protein. They are found in high levels in animal foods like liver, sardines, sweetbreads, turkey, anchovies, and are also found in asparagus and mushrooms.

Purine-restricted diets—used in the past as a primary treatment of gout and uric acid kidney stone formation—are now considered an adjunct to medication for these conditions.

PYRIDOXINE is the chemical name for vitamin B_6.

See Vitamin B_6

R

RDA, Recommended Dietary Allowances, are estimates, based on available scientific knowledge, of the amounts of nutrients that population groups should consume over a period of time. The recommendations are not requirements for individuals, but are planned to meet the needs of groups of healthy people over a period of time. The RDA's are not intended to be used to evaluate an individual's food intake, but they are sometimes used for this. The recommendations are not averages, except for energy (Calories), but are calculated for persons with the highest requirements. That's why for all nutrients listed, except Calories, recommendations are greater than most healthy people need. This means you don't have to take in, every day, all of the quantities listed for each nutrient in order to be well nourished. Many authorities feel two thirds or more of the RDA is adequate for most. The RDA's also do not take into account special needs persons may have because of diseases, inherited metabolic disorders or infections.

Except for energy (Calories), all other allowances lump together in one group all people aged 51 and over.

We are currently using the 1980 revision of the RDA which consists of three tables. This is the ninth revision of the RDA.

See U.S. RDA

REFINED refers to the process by which the chaff, bran and germ are removed from a cereal grain, leaving only the endosperm. White flour is made from the endosperm of wheat. The major criticism of refined flour and cereal products is that they are made up predominantly of starch and are low in many nutrients normally found in the germ and bran portion of the grain.

See Whole grain

RETINOL is the natural form of vitamin A found in animal tissue. In all animals and humans it is found mainly in the liver with lesser amounts in the kidney, lung and fat tissue. Approximately one-third of the necessary vitamin A is supplied in the animal form, retinol.

See Vitamin A

RIBOFLAVIN is the chemical name for vitamin B_2.

See Vitamin B_2

ROCALTROL, *see* Calcitriol

ROSE HIPS are the red fruits formed at the base of rose flowers. They are one of the richest natural sources of vitamin C. Rose hips are made into a vitamin-rich syrup, brewed into tea and used as an ingredient in vitamin C supplements. Vitamin tablets con-

Recommended Daily Dietary Allowancesᵃ

	Age (years)	Weight (kg)	Weight (lbs)	Height (cm)	Height (in)	Protein (g)	Vitamin A (µg R.E.)ᵇ	Vitamin D (µg)ᶜ	Vitamin E (mg α T.E.)ᵈ	Vitamin C (mg)	Thiamin (mg)	Riboflavin (mg)	Niacin (mg N.E.)ᵉ	Vitamin B₆ (mg)	Folacin (µg)	Vitamin B₁₂ (µg)	Calcium (mg)	Phosphorus (mg)	Magnesium (mg)	Iron (mg)	Zinc (mg)	Iodine (µg)
Infants	0.0–0.5	6	13	60	24	kg×2.2	420	10	3	35	0.3	0.4	6	0.3	30	0.5ᵃ	360	240	50	10	3	40
	0.5–1.0	9	20	71	28	kg×2.0	400	10	4	35	0.5	0.6	8	0.6	45	1.5	540	360	70	15	5	50
Children	1–3	13	29	90	35	23	400	10	5	45	0.7	0.8	9	0.9	100	2.0	800	800	150	15	10	70
	4–6	20	44	112	44	30	500	10	6	45	0.9	1.0	11	1.3	200	2.5	800	800	200	10	10	90
	7–10	28	62	132	52	34	700	10	7	45	1.2	1.4	16	1.6	300	3.0	800	800	250	10	10	120
Males	11–14	45	99	157	62	45	1000	10	8	50	1.4	1.6	18	1.8	400	3.0	1200	1200	350	18	15	150
	15–18	66	145	176	69	56	1000	10	10	60	1.4	1.7	18	2.0	400	3.0	1200	1200	400	18	15	150
	19–22	70	154	177	70	56	1000	7.5	10	60	1.5	1.7	19	2.2	400	3.0	800	800	350	10	15	150
	23–50	70	154	178	70	56	1000	5	10	60	1.4	1.6	18	2.2	400	3.0	800	800	350	10	15	150
	51+	70	154	178	70	56	1000	5	10	60	1.2	1.4	16	2.2	400	3.0	800	800	350	10	15	150
Females	11–14	46	101	157	62	46	800	10	8	50	1.1	1.3	15	1.8	400	3.0	1200	1200	300	18	15	150
	15–18	55	120	163	64	46	800	10	8	60	1.1	1.3	14	2.0	400	3.0	1200	1200	300	18	15	150
	19–22	55	120	163	64	44	800	7.5	8	60	1.1	1.3	14	2.0	400	3.0	800	800	300	18	15	150
	23–50	55	120	163	64	44	800	5	8	60	1.0	1.2	13	2.0	400	3.0	800	800	300	18	15	150
	51+	55	120	163	64	44	800	5	8	60	1.0	1.2	13	2.0	400	3.0	800	800	300	10	15	150
Pregnancy						+30	+200	+5	+2	+20	+0.4	+0.3	+2	+0.6	+400	+1.0	+400	+400	+150	h	+5	+25
Lactating						+20	+400	+5	+3	+40	+0.5	+0.5	+5	+0.5	+100	+1.0	+400	+400	+150	h	+10	+50

[a] The allowances are intended to provide for individual variations among most normal persons as they live in the United States under usual environmental stresses. Diets should be based on a variety of common foods in order to provide other nutrients for which human requirements have been less well defined. See p. 227 for heights, weights and recommended intake.

[b] Retinol equivalents. 1 Retinol equivalent = 1 μg retinol or 6 μg β carotene.

[c] As cholecalciferol. 10 μg cholecalciferol = 400 IU vitamin D.

[d] α-tocopherol equivalents. 1 mg d-α-tocopherol = 1 α T.E.

[e] 1 N.E. (niacin equivalent) is equal to 1 mg of niacin or 60 mg of dietary tryptophan.

[f] The folacin allowances refer to dietary sources as determined by *Lactobacillus casei* assay after treatment with enzymes ("conjugases") to make polyglutamyl forms of the vitamin available to the test organism.

[g] The RDA for vitamin B_{12} in infants is based on average concentration of the vitamin in human milk. The allowances after weaning are based on energy intake (as recommended by the American Academy of Pediatrics) and consideration of other factors such as intestinal absorption.

[h] The increased requirement during pregnancy cannot be met by the iron content of habitual American diets nor by the existing iron stores of many women; therefore the use of 30–60 mg of supplemental iron is recommended. Iron needs during lactation are not substantially different from those of non-pregnant women, but continued supplementation of the mother for 2–3 months after parturition is advisable in order to replenish stores depleted by pregnancy.

Source: Food and Nutrition Board, National Academy of Sciences—National Research Council.

Recommended Dietary Allowances, Revised 1980

Estimated Safe and Adequate Daily Dietary Intakes of Selected Vitamins and Minerals[a]

	Age (years)	VITAMINS			TRACE ELEMENTS[b]						ELECTROLYTES		
		Vitamin K (µg)	Biotin (µg)	Pantothenic Acid (mg)	Copper (mg)	Manganese (mg)	Fluoride (mg)	Chromium (mg)	Selenium (mg)	Molybdenum (mg)	Sodium (mg)	Potassium (mg)	Chloride (mg)
Infants	0-0.5	12	35	2	0.5-0.7	0.5-0.7	0.1-0.5	0.01-0.04	0.01-0.04	0.03-0.06	115-350	350-925	275-700
	0.5-1	10-20	50	3	0.7-1.0	0.7-1.0	0.2-1.0	0.02-0.06	0.02-0.06	0.04-0.08	250-750	425-1275	400-1200
Children	1-3	15-30	65	3	1.0-1.5	1.0-1.5	0.5-1.5	0.02-0.08	0.02-0.08	0.05-0.1	325-975	550-1650	500-1500
and	4-6	20-40	85	3-4	1.5-2.0	1.5-2.0	1.0-2.5	0.03-0.12	0.03-0.12	0.06-0.15	450-1350	775-2325	700-2100
Adolescents	7-10	30-60	120	4-5	2.0-2.5	2.0-3.0	1.5-2.5	0.05-0.2	0.05-0.2	0.1-0.3	600-1800	1000-3000	925-2775
	11+	50-100	100-200	4-7	2.0-3.0	2.5-5.0	1.5-2.5	0.05-0.2	0.05-0.2	0.15-0.5	900-2700	1525-4575	1400-4200
Adults		70-140	100-200	4-7	2.0-3.0	2.5-5.0	1.5-4.0	0.05-0.2	0.05-0.2	0.15-0.5	1100-3300	1875-5625	1700-5100

[a] Because there is less information on which to base allowances, these figures are not given in the main table of the RDA and are provided here in the form of ranges of recommended intakes.

[b] Since the toxic levels for many trace elements may be only several times usual intakes, the upper levels for the trace elements given in this table should not be habitually exceeded.

Mean Heights and Weights and Recommended Energy Intake[a] Recommended Dietary Allowances. Revised 1980

Category	Age (years)	Weight (kg)	Weight (lb)	Height (cm)	Height (in)	Energy Needs (with range) (kcal)	(MJ)
Infants	0.0–0.5	6	13	60	24	kg × 115 (95–145)	kg × .48
	0.5–1.0	9	20	71	28	kg × 105 (80–135)	kg × .44
Children	1–3	13	29	90	35	1300 (900–1800)	5.5
	4–6	20	44	112	44	1700 (1300–2300)	7.1
	7–10	28	62	132	52	2400 (1650–3300)	10.1
Males	11–14	45	99	157	62	2700 (2000–3700)	11.3
	15–18	66	145	176	69	2800 (2100–3900)	11.8
	19–22	70	154	177	70	2900 (2500–3300)	12.2
	23–50	70	154	178	70	2700 (2300–3100)	11.3
	51–75	70	154	178	70	2400 (2000–2800)	10.1
	76+	70	154	178	70	2050 (1650–2450)	8.6
Females	11–14	46	101	157	62	2200 (1500–3000)	9.2
	15–18	55	120	163	64	2100 (1200–3000)	8.8
	19–22	55	120	163	64	2100 (1700–2500)	8.8

Category	Age (years)	Weight (kg)	(lb)	Height (cm)	(in)	Energy Needs (with range) (kcal)		(MJ)
Females	23–50	55	120	163	64	2000	(1600–2400)	8.4
	51–75	55	120	163	64	1800	(1400–2200)	7.6
	76+	55	120	163	64	1600	(1200–2000)	6.7
Pregnancy						+300		
Lactation						+500		

[a]The data in this table have been assembled from the observed median heights and weights of children shown in Table 1, together with desirable weights for adults given in Table 2 for the mean heights of men (70 inches) and women (64 inches) between the ages of 18 and 34 years as surveyed in the U.S. population (HEW/NCHS data).

The energy allowances for the young adults are for men and women doing light work. The allowances for the two older groups represent mean energy needs over these age spans, allowing for a 2% decrease in basal (resting) metabolic rate per decade and a reduction in activity of 200 kcal/day for men and women between 51 and 75 years, 500 kcal for men over 75 years and 400 kcal for women over 75. The customary range of daily energy output is shown for adults in parentheses, and is based on a variation in energy needs of ± 400 kcal at any one age, emphasizing the wide range of energy intakes appropriate for any group of people.

Energy allowances for children through age 18 are based on median energy intakes of children of these ages followed in longitudinal growth studies. The values in parentheses are 10th and 90th percentiles of energy intake, to indicate the range of energy consumption among children of these ages.

Source: Food and Nutrition Board, National Academy of Sciences—National Research Council.

228

taining only rose hips as the vitamin C source would be too large to swallow. Supplements labeled *Rose Hips Vitamin C* contain only about 2 percent of the vitamin from rose hips; the remainder often is synthetic Vitamin C.

See Vitamin C

ROUGHAGE, *see* Fiber

S

POCKET ENCYCLOPEDIA OF NUTRITION 229

bringing out, rinse them in the Vitamin C source as well as too large a workdilico ated and the Botanic oil and how high the most common ulilar and so on because of their Vitamin effort boo limp the Bramotes often is equaling. We Bram.

SACCHARIN, *see* Artificial sweeteners

SALT, or sodium chloride (NaC1), is a combination of the metal sodium and the gas chlorine, used as a seasoning and preservative. Both components are essential elements in the body but there is not likely to be a deficiency of either as most Americans eat much more, by about ten times, than recommended amounts. The body adjusts to high and low intakes up to a point.

Excess salt intake over many years may be a factor in the development of high blood pressure in people who are susceptible. Salt can also pose a problem for people with kidney disease or when the body has adapted to a low-salt diet. These people should read food labels carefully to avoid salt and sodium-containing food additives, like MSG (monosodium glutamate).

See Hypertension, Sodium

SALT SUBSTITUTES are seasonings used instead of regular table salt. Salt is 40 percent sodium and 60 percent chloride. One teaspoon of regular salt contains 2,300 milligrams of sodium. A salt substitute may have all of the sodium removed, replaced by potassium. This type of salt substitute would be a potassium chloride salt. It has a bitter aftertaste and is not acceptable to all people. Persons with a heart condition should check with their doctor before switching to a potassium chloride salt substitute. Potassium is involved with the normal functioning of the heart and too much can be as dangerous as too little. "Lite" salts are salt substitutes in which part of the sodium is replaced by potassium, partially reducing the sodium in the salt. These salt substitutes are sodium chloride and potassium chloride. Morton "Lite" Salt is a brand-name example of this type of salt substitute. It has only 975 milligrams of sodium in a teaspoon.

Another type of salt substitute are saltless seasoning mixtures. *Mrs. Dash* is a brand-name example of an herb and spice blend that can be used in place of salt. Following is a homemade version of a saltless seasoning mixture:

Saltless Seasoning "Salt"

½ teaspoon garlic powder
¼ teaspoon powdered thyme
½ teaspoon onion powder
½ teaspoon paprika
¼ teaspoon ground celery seed
½ teaspoon pepper
½ teaspoon dry mustard

Combine; store in a closed container in a dry place.

SALT TABLETS are used to replace salt loss in excessive, prolonged sweating. However, water replacement for sweat loss is more important than salt replacement because during perspiration water loss is greater than salt loss. Normally, salt in foods can replace losses from perspiration but if more than 5 to 7 pounds of sweat is lost during one to two days of heat exposure, salt tablets may be needed. Salt tablets should be used only under a doctor's guidance and the use should be short term. Currently athletes no longer use salt tablets. Instead, they eat salty foods for twenty-four hours after an endurance event.

SATURATED FATS are found in meat, fish, poultry, eggs and dairy products. Animal fat tends to be saturated but exceptions are poultry fat and cod liver oil, both of which contain a lot of unsaturated fat.

Vegetable oils are low in saturated fats except for coconut, cocoa butter and palm oil.

See Fat, Heart disease, Monounsaturated fats, Polyunsaturated fats

SCURVY is a disease caused by a severe deficiency of vitamin C. As little as 10 mg a day will protect against it. Diseases resembling scurvy were described in writings as early as 1,550 B.C. Sailors on long sea voyages often developed scurvy because fresh fruits were not eaten on the ships. The use of lemons and limes to prevent scurvy among British sailors was the basis for their nickname, "limeys."

Scurvy is not common in the United States but is seen in some babies in the second half of their first year. It is even less common in adults.

Pain, tenderness and swelling of thighs and legs and bone deformities are common symptoms of scurvy in infants. The baby is also pale, irritable and cries when handled. If the baby has teeth, the gums will be swollen and bleeding.

In adults, scurvy symptoms are blood spots on the

skin, anemia, swelling, infection and bleeding of gums with loose teeth. Slight injury causes bruises.

Scurvy responds within a few days to doses of 100 to 200 mg tablets of vitamin C. About two cups of orange juice will provide an equivalent amount of the vitamin. Anemia and bone deformities will take longer to reverse.

SEA SALT is often touted as being healthier than regular salt. In fact they are practically the same. Both must contain at least 97.5 percent sodium chloride to be labeled salt and therefore both are extremely high sources of sodium. If you are on a low-salt diet you must limit sea salt as well as regular salt.

Sea salt contains magnesium and calcium but the amounts are so small they are insignificant. The iodine originally found in sea salt is lost as the salt is evaporated from sea water.

SELENIUM is an essential mineral needed in very small amounts. Some selenium is found in all body tissues with most in the kidney, liver, spleen, pancreas and testicles. Selenium functions with vitamin E as an antioxidant, preventing cell damage from peroxidized (degraded) fats. It also protects against toxic substances like arsenic and mercury. Deficiencies of the mineral are not easy to detect because vitamin E and sulfur-containing amino acids can substitute for selenium in some of its functions.

The estimated safe and adequate intake ranges from 0.05 to 0.2 mg a day for people over age 7. For younger children 0.01 to 0.12 mg is suggested. Diets in the United States usually provide from 0.05 to 0.2 mg a day. Meat and fish are rich sources. The amount of selenium in grains and cereals depends on the level of the mineral in the soil where they were grown. High-protein foods are usually high in selenium.

Some studies suggest that selenium may have anti-cancer properties and that selenium deficiency may contribute to heart disease and cataract formation. As too much selenium can be poisonous, if any supplements are taken, they should contain no more than the estimated safe range indicated above.

See Minerals

SEROTONIN, *see* Tryptophan

SET POINT refers to the weight that is most comfortable or natural for the body. A person usually stays at or around this weight. Some people have a higher set point than others of similar height, explaining the varying weights for a given height. The set point theory states that it is hard for a person to reset the natural set point and lower their weight. According to this theory, weight loss is doomed to fail if the person wants to become thinner than their natural set point. It may be possible, however, to readjust the set point downward by regular exercise.

See Diet

SNACKS have traditionally been defined as those foods eaten between meals. Today, however, many people eat more snacks than actual meals so it may be appropriate to redefine "snacking" as eating small amounts of foods at any time during the day. Snack foods are often associated with foods high in fat, salt and sugar and low in nutrients. This need not be the case as any food can be a "snack." Those who snack frequently, rather than eating traditional meals, need to make a more conscious effort to select nutritious snack foods—yogurt, fruit, cheese, juice, raw vegetables, nuts and dried fruit are all good choices.

Tips for Sensible Snacking

• Snack only when you are hungry, not because some outside cue is tempting you to eat.

• Control the size of snacks. Buy dixie cups of ice cream rather than spooning your portion from a half gallon. Get individual bags of pretzels and chips rather than a larger bag. Buy muffins or cupcakes rather than a cake. Eat bite-sized candy bars.

• Make snacks count. Think of them as additions to meals. If you had a burger and fries for lunch, make your mid-afternoon snack fresh fruit. If you had time only for coffee before work, try orange juice and a muffin on your coffee break. Plan an after-dinner snack—for example, save your salad to eat in front of the TV.

• Plan each snack to give you a nutrient bonus. Citrus fruits provide vitamin C. Cheese, yogurt and ice cream are sources of calcium. Raw vegetables offer vitamins, minerals and fiber.

• Keep salty, heavily sweetened or fried snacks for occasional use; they are high in calories and low in nutrients.

• Never feel obligated to eat just because someone offers you a snack. Club soda or mineral water and a wedge of lemon or lime is a zero-calorie alternative to snacking.

SODA is also referred to as "soda pop," "pop," or "soft drinks," while "hard" drinks refer to alcohol. Soda is usually, but not always, carbonated, contains a sweetening agent, edible acids, natural or artificial flavors and colors; many contain caffeine. Soda is the most popular beverage in the United States. In 1983 Americans averaged forty gallons per person, surpassing milk, coffee and beer, which placed second, third and fourth respectively. Soda accounts for 25 percent of our refined sugar intake and provides about 8 percent of our daily calories. Most soft drinks are basically sugared, flavored water supplying approximately 150 Calories in 12 ounces (1 can), with only trace amounts of other nutrients.

The first soda was sold in 1772 but it did not become popular until the mid 1800s. Late in the nineteenth century a druggist named Pemberton created a soft drink made from the extract of *cocoa* and the extract of the African *kola* nut. Around the same time another druggist named Hires introduced bottled root beer. Today every conceivable flavor soft drink has been introduced but cola, ginger ale, lemon-lime, orange, root beer and grape remain the favorites. To ensure continued popularity and continued consumption of soda, advertisers spend over $200 million each year to convince the public that it's "the real thing."

See Caffeine, Diet sodas

SODIUM is an essential element that helps maintain water balance, acid-base balance and also functions in absorption and transport of nutrients, muscle contraction, electrical transmission of nerve signals and influences the permeability of cell membranes.

We eat from three to seven grams (3,000 to 7,000 mg) of sodium a day, while a daily intake of 500 mg should meet the body's need. It is estimated that people lose from 40 to 220 mg a day in urine, feces and sweat. Each person's actual need depends on the amount of work they do and the climate they live in because sodium is lost in sweat. Sodium intake depends on eating habits.

Sodium is in most foods, either naturally or added during processing or in cooking. It is not always easy to tell which foods contain a lot of sodium. Artichokes, celery, carrots, greens, spinach, egg white, milk, beets and white turnips are foods naturally high in sodium. Fruits, coffee, tea, jelly, shredded wheat, puffed rice, fresh fish, rice, pasta and oatmeal are low. Water in many areas contains significant amounts of sodium and

Sodium Content of Common Foods

Food	Sodium (mg)	Portion
Corn, fresh	1	1 ear
Peanuts	1	4 tbs
Oatmeal, regular, cooked, no salt added	1	¾ cup
Pineapple, canned	1	1 slice
Butter, sweet	2	1 tbsp
Coffee	2	6 ounces
Herb-Ox Low-Sodium Beef Broth	9	1 packet
Celery, raw	25	1 stalk
Campbell's Low-Sodium Corn Soup	30	10¾ ounces
Carrots, raw	34	1 medium
Saltine	35	1 cracker
Butter, salted	50	1 tbsp
Chicken	57	3 ounces
Fudge	60	1 ounce
Egg	70	1 medium
Graham cracker	95	1 large
Peas, frozen	106	½ cup
Pepperidge Farm White Bread	117	2 slices
Whole milk	130	1 cup
Planters Cocktail Peanuts	132	1 ounce
White bread	140	1 slice
Heinz Tomato Ketchup	154	1 tbsp
Skippy Creamy Peanut Butter	167	2 tbsp
Lay's Potato Chips	191	1 ounce
Worcestershire Sauce	206	1 tbsp
Kraft American Cheese	238	1 slice (1 oz)
Kellogg's Corn Flakes	260	1 ounce
Peanuts, salted	275	¼ cup
Taco Bell Bean Burrito	288	Entire serving

Food	Sodium (mg)	Portion
Campbell's Tomato Juice	292	4 ounces
Oscar Mayer Bacon	302	3 slices
Wish-Bone Italian Salad Dressing	315	1 tbsp
Tomato juice	320	½ cup
Del Monte Sweet Peas, canned	349	½ cup
Beef	381	3 ounces
Jell-O Chocolate Instant Pudding	404	½ cup
Devil's food pudding cake mix	435	¹⁄₁₂ of a cake
Frankfurter	495	1
English muffin, buttered	466	Entire muffin
Oscar Mayer Bologna	672	3 slices
Burger King Whaler	735	Entire serving
Herb-Ox Instant Beef Broth	818	1 packet
Burger King Whopper	909	Entire serving
Campbell's Beans & Franks	958	8 ounces
Heinz dill pickles	1,137	1 large pickle
Swanson Fried Chicken Dinner	1,152	Complete dinner
Chef Boy-Ar-Dee Beefaroni	1,186	8 ounces
Soy sauce	1,320	1 tbsp
McDonald's Big Mac	1,510	Entire serving
Kentucky Fried Chicken dinner, extra crispy	1,915	Dinner for 1 person
Kentucky Fried Chicken dinner, original recipe dinner	2,285	Dinner for 1 person

Foods naturally high in sodium

Artichokes	Greens	Milk
Celery	Spinach	Beets
Carrots	Egg white	White turnip

Foods naturally low in sodium

Fruits	Shredded wheat	Rice
Coffee and tea	Puffed rice	Pasta
Jelly	Fresh fish	Oatmeal

sometimes sodium is added to water through the use of water softeners.

It is not generally agreed that sodium causes high blood pressure for all persons. There is agreement, however, on the view that sodium reduction can't hurt and may prevent high blood pressure in some people.

See Salt

SODIUM BICARBONATE, or baking soda, acts as a buffer in the body to maintain neutrality and ensure normal body function. It is used as an antacid (Alka-Seltzer) which should be avoided by people on a low-salt diet as it is high in sodium.

Baking soda is also used as a leavening agent in baked goods either alone or as an ingredient of baking powder. Baking soda is also used as a home remedy for indigestion; this, too, should be avoided by persons on low-salt diets.

See Antacids

SORBITOL is a naturally occurring sugar alcohol found in berries, cherries, plums, pears, apples and blackstrap molasses. It is 60 percent as sweet as table sugar (sucrose). Commercially, sorbitol is used as an additive in "sugarless" or "sugar-free" foods. This is somewhat misleading since sorbitol contains the same number of calories as sugar but it is handled differently by the body. It is burned in the body to produce carbon dioxide and never appears in the blood as glucose the way other sugars do. Eating large amounts of sorbitol can cause diarrhea.

See Mannitol

SOUR CREAM is a pasteurized, homogenized cream cultured with bacteria *(Streptococcus lactos)* resulting in a gel. It contains 18 to 20 percent fat. One tablespoon of sour cream equals 20 Calories.

SOYBEANS are one of the world's most important oilseed crops and a staple food in the Orient. Soybeans were first grown in China, long before written history. They were introduced to the United States in the early 1800s but major cultivation as a cash crop did not begin until the 1930s. Today the United States is the world's largest supplier of soybeans and soybean oil is our largest single source of vegetable oil.

Soybeans contain 30 to 50 percent protein, 14 to 24 percent carbohydrate and 13 to 25 percent oil, which is high in polyunsaturated fatty acids. Soybeans are a good source of calcium as well as being rich in many other vitamins and minerals. The quality of the protein in soybeans is close to meat, fish and poultry, making it an excellent protein replacement or protein extender.

In Asia, soybeans—in various forms from soy milk to deep-fried mature soybeans—are a regular part of the diet. In the United States more soy is used for animal feed than for human foods. Food manufacturers, however, are increasingly using more soybeans in the development of new food products.

Below is a listing of some of the uses for soybeans.

PRODUCT	DESCRIPTION	USES
Soybeans	Whole soybeans	In recipes like other dried beans or roasted as a snack food
		When immature, as a hot vegetable
Ketjap	A type of soy sauce	A flavoring agent
Miso	A fermented food paste the consistency of peanut butter, made from rice, salt and soybeans	A flavoring added to soups and vegetables or served over pasta; miso originated in China and is used widely in Japan
Soybean flour (soy flour)	Finely ground soybeans	A protein extender in bakery products, meat products, breakfast cereals, infant foods, desserts
Soybean lecithin	A fatlike substance removed from the oil during processing	An antioxidant, emulsifier and softener in food manufacturing
Soybean milk	A beverage resulting from soaking and grinding soybeans	The base for soy-based infant formulas
		The base for making tofu
Soybean oil	Oil extract of soybeans	In margarine, cooking oil and salad dressing
Soy protein concentrates and isolates	Extracted soybean protein	A protein extender in all varieties of processed foods
Soy sauce (Shoyu or Chaing-yu	Liquid resulting from fermented soybeans	A flavoring agent that has been used in China for 2,500 years

PRODUCT	DESCRIPTION	USES
Tempeh	A mold-fermented Indonesian food	A main dish; the mold starter makes it a good source of vitamin B_{12}
Textured soybeans	Meat analogs: baconlike bits, simulated sausages, ham, chicken and bacon slices	A vegetable protein substitute for meat
Tofu (Sofu)	Coagulated soybean milk	A soft cheeselike curd, eaten as a substitute for meat; contains 53 percent protein, 26 percent fat, 17 percent carbohydrate and 4 percent fiber
Tofutti	Nondairy frozen, ice cream-like dessert made from tofu	An ice cream substitute; it is high in fat, calories and protein but free of cholesterol and lactose (milk sugar)

SOY MILK is a mixture of water, soybeans, vegetable oil and some other ingredients such as kelp, pearl barley, barley malt and salt. While it is a nutritious drink, it should not be used as the sole food for infants. It is not the same as soy-based infant formulas which are specially made to meet all the infant's nutritional needs.

Soy milk has the same amount of protein as cow's milk and only one third the amount of fat. Most of this fat is unsaturated. Unlike cow's milk it is a poor source of calcium. Some soy milks are vitamin B_{12} fortified.

See Soy

SPIRULINIA, a type of blue-green algae, is sold as a food supplement in powder or pill form. Spirulinia can be a source of protein, vitamins and minerals, but there are insignificant levels of these nutrients in the amounts normally used. Spirulinia has been touted as an aid to weight loss because of its phenylalanine content which is supposed to switch off hunger pangs. There is no scientific basis to these claims, however. Phenylalanine is an amino acid found in most proteins.

Spirulinia and other algae contain large amounts of uric acid forming nucleic acids. If eaten in excess they could cause kidney stones or gout in susceptible people.

See Gout, Kidney stones

SPORTS DRINKS are fluid, calorie and nutrient replacement beverages used by athletes to replace fluids and nutrients which are used up during exercise and lost in sweat. Plain water is probably the best drink after strenuous exercise; if a sports drink is preferred, experts recommend that it be diluted with water so the athlete does not get too high a concentration of sugar, which will draw water into the intestines and dehydrate the body. Although the minerals added to sports drinks are not harmful, they are not really needed, as normal eating will replace a wider variety of lost minerals within the next day or two.

See Gatorade

SPORTS NUTRITION is a growing area of specialty

that focuses on the needs of the amateur and professional athlete to maximize strength and endurance through proper nutrition. Many athletes believe they need more protein to build and increase muscle mass. Many experiments have confirmed that added protein does not build muscles and does not increase strength, endurance or speed.

What the athlete does need is added fuel (Calories) to see him through training and the actual event. Protein can be burned for calories but this is both an expensive and inefficient energy source. A mixture of carbohydrate and fat calories with adequate protein is a more appropriate diet plan. Short duration, high intensity activities—for example, a high jump or 100 yard swim—depend mainly on carbohydrate for fuel. Long duration, endurance activities, such as marathon races, also depend on carbohydrate energy, especially the storage form of carbohydrate called gycogen found in the muscles. These long-duration athletes also utilize body fat stores to make it through the grueling activity. Low-carbohydrate, high-fat, high-protein diets have actually been shown to hamper the athlete's ability to perform.

Whenever energy intake and energy use is high, extra B vitamins are needed. If the extra energy is provided in the form of nourishing foods, these foods will provide additional B vitamins as well. Supplemental vitamins are not automatically needed.

See Gatorade, Glycogen loading

SPRUE, *see* Celiac disease

STARCH BLOCKER is a protein made from beans (e.g., kidney, northern or others) which blocks the digestion of starch by interfering with the action of an enzyme (alpha-amylase). It was recommended as an aid for weight control. Available in pill form, it was claimed that each pill blocked the digestion of approximately 400 to 750 starch Calories. A low calorie diet (1,200 Calories) was suggested along with the starch blockers which in itself could cause weight loss.

Users of the pills complain of nausea, vomiting, diarrhea, gas and abdominal pain. In response to these reports the Food and Drug Administration in 1982 banned sales of the product until it could be proved safe and effective.

STONES, *see* Calculi

STRESS VITAMINS usually contain a mixture of B vitamins and vitamin C. While there have been reports that extra vitamin C is helpful in some physical stress conditions like burns, surgery, injuries and infection, there is no real evidence that added vitamins can help a person handle emotional and/or mental stress. Not much research has focused on this type of stress.

During stressful times a regular, not high potency, multivitamin supplement and a little extra vitamin C may be helpful. At worst it will do no harm. Exercise is also a great stress reliever. Eating well is important; overeating is a bad idea since stress slows down the production of digestive enzymes and this could lead to indigestion.

SUCROSE is more commonly known as table sugar, which is refined from the sugar beet or sugar cane. It is broken down in the digestive tract to two simpler sugars—glucose and fructose. It is estimated that we eat over 125 pounds of sweeteners per person per year. More than half of this is sucrose.

SUCROSE POLYESTER, or SPE, is an artificial fat manufactured by replacing the glycerol portion of the triglyceride molecule with sucrose. The result is a molecule with three fatty acids bound to a sucrose backbone. This substance has all the cooking and eating qualities of traditional fats but it cannot be digested or absorbed because of its molecular structure. Since it cannot be utilized by the body, it yields no calories for energy. In addition, in the gut it exhibits an affinity for fatlike compounds such as cholesterol, binding to them and carrying them out of the body through the stool. This prevents their buildup in the blood.

Though still in the experimental stage, sucrose polyester has potential as a food additive which will aid in the treatment of obesity and cardiovascular disease. Some negative side effects to the substance are loose, oily stools, decrease in absorption of fat-soluble vitamins and possible lowering effect of HDL cholesterol.

SUGAR, a sweet-tasting substance available in granulated, powdered, liquid or cube forms, is made from sugar beets or sugar cane. Americans eat about 75 pounds of sugar a year, but when other sweeteners like corn syrup are added in, the total of sugars and sweeteners averages about 125 pounds.

Sugar is a source of energy—about 16 Calories for each teaspoon and little else. Sugar is considered to be a factor in dental decay and because it tastes good it may encourage people to eat more calories than they need. Other charges—that sugar causes hyperactivity in children, diabetes or heart disease—are not supported by scientific evidence.

On a food label sugar may appear as dextrose, fructose, corn syrup, corn sweeteners, lactose, brown sugar, honey or molasses.

See Carbohydrates

SULFITES like potassium and sodium meta-bisulfite, sulfur dioxide, sodium sulfite, sodium and potassium bisulfite, are preservatives used to eliminate bacteria, preserve freshness and brightness, prevent browning, increase storage life and prevent spoilage of certain foods. Sulfiting agents are used on fresh fruits and vegetables, dried fruits, processed potatoes, shrimp and to improve the quality and texture of wines and baked products. Washing the food does not remove the sulfiting agent.

Sulfites have caused acute asthma attacks in people who are sensitive to them. They have been linked to thirteen deaths and to health problems in more than 500 others. Reactions range from nausea and diarrhea to hives, shortness of breath and fatal shock.

In 1985, the Food and Drug Administration (FDA) revoked the GRAS (Generally Recognized As Safe) status of sulfites for use on fruits and vegetables intended to be sold or served raw. In August 1986, the FDA banned the use of sulfites on fresh vegetables and fruits in retail sale in food stores and restaurants.

Sulfites are also found in some asthma medications. The FDA has proposed requiring a warning statement for all prescription drugs containing sulfites. This will enable physicians to avoid prescribing drugs containing sulfites to patients that are sensitive to them.

See GRAS

SULFUR is an essential mineral found in every cell of the body. There are about 175 gm of sulfur in an adult's body. It is found in two vitamins—biotin and B_1 (thiamin)—and in three amino acids. Sulfur is in skin, nails and hair and is sometimes called a "beauty mineral" because it is believed to keep hair shiny and skin clear. Sulfur functions in body metabolism and combines with toxic substances so they can be passed out safely in the urine.

There are no recommended levels of intake for sulfur because when protein intake is adequate, sulfur is too.

Proteins in food contain an average of one percent sulfur. Good food sources are cheese, eggs, fish, grains, dried peas and beans, poultry and nuts.

See Minerals

SUNSHINE VITAMIN, *see* Vitamin D.

T

TANNINS are a group of chemicals which occur naturally in many plants and contribute to the astringent taste of these foods. Some of the taste of coffee and tea comes from tannins. It is believed that they may help to stop common diarrhea and for that reason weak, sweetened tea is often recommended as a replacement fluid for those with diarrhea.

TARDIVE DYSKINESIA, *see* Choline

TARTRAZINE, *see* Artificial colors, Food allergies, MSG

TASTE BUDS are chemical receptors in the mouth, mostly on the tongue but also on the inner cheeks, palate, epiglottis and pharynx (upper part of the throat). The average person has 12,000 taste buds and

249

can sense four types of taste: salty, throughout the mouth; sweet, at the tip of the tongue; bitter, at the back of the mouth; and sour, on the sides of the mouth. Taste buds are excited by the chemical substances we eat, sending sensations to the brain. Young children have very acute taste buds which often accounts for their rejection of certain foods; the taste they perceive is more intense than would be sensed by an adult. As we age our sense of taste diminishes. Salty is the most persistent of our taste sensations and the last to fade. Medications, diseases and medical treatments like chemotherapy can interfere with our sense of taste.

TEA is the most popular beverage in the world, second only to water. Quenching, comforting and aromatic, tea was discovered, legend has it, nearly 5,000 years ago, when some leaves of the camellia drifted into the kettle of the Emperor Shen Nung of China. The beverage moved across the Orient to the Japanese, who elevated it to a ceremonial tradition. Tea did not reach Europe until the early 1600s, where it was very expensive and available only to those of great wealth. Tea caddies were designed with locks to hold this precious substance and for many years in England tea was weighed for sale on the same exacting scales used to make up drug prescriptions.

Tea did not come to the new world with the early colonists; it was too expensive and rare. By the time of the Revolutionary War, however, tea had become a popular drink. Everyone is familiar with the famous Boston Tea Party, when the American colonists dumped 342 chests of tea into Boston Harbor to protest English taxes. After the colonies became independent, tea played a large role in growing American trade. Clipper ships were first designed in the hope of finding a faster way to transport tea across oceans.

Until the 1904 St. Louis World Fair, Americans drank tea hot. An inventive salesman, unable to sell tea on a hot day, put ice in it. To this day, the United States and Canada are the only countries in the world that use "iced" tea regularly.

Without cream and sugar, tea offers little except a few calories and a source of fluoride. Green tea is a good source of vitamin K. A cup of tea has about half the caffeine content of a cup of coffee, 30 to 60 mg a cup depending on the strength of the brew.

Tea is the leaf of an Oriental evergreen. The word has evolved, however, to have several other meanings: a hot beverage made from herbs, spices or flowers (no actual tea leaves are in these mixtures); an afternoon or early evening meal in Britain; or a large morning or afternoon reception.

Our major supplier of tea is Sri Lanka; India is the number one supplier in the world. Basically there are three types of tea. Black tea is fermented, dried tea leaves. Oolong tea is semi-fermented, dried tea leaves. Green tea is steamed and dried tea leaves; the steaming process prevents fermentation. Research has shown that green tea can lower serum cholesterol in those who use it regularly.

See Herbal tea

TEMPERATURE is measured according to three scales: Celsius (Centigrade), Fahrenheit and Kelvin (Absolute). The scientific community tends to use the Centigrade scale, the medical and general public use the Fahrenheit scale, and the Kelvin scale is used in inhalation therapy. The following shows a comparison of the three systems of measurement.

See Body temperature, Calories

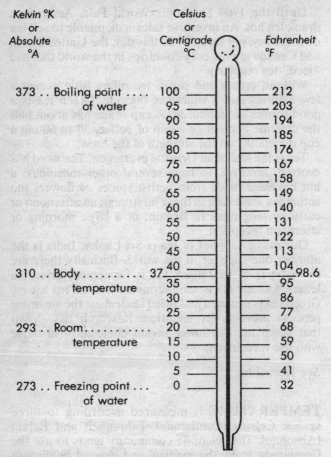

Kelvin °K or Absolute °A	Celsius or Centigrade °C	Fahrenheit °F
373 .. Boiling point .... of water	100	212
	95	203
	90	194
	85	185
	80	176
	75	167
	70	158
	65	149
	60	140
	55	131
	50	122
	45	113
310 .. Body .... temperature	37 40	104 98.6
	35	95
	30	86
	25	77
293 .. Room .... temperature	20	68
	15	59
	10	50
	5	41
273 .. Freezing point ... of water	0	32

THIAMIN is the chemical name for vitamin B_1. Thiamin may also be spelled "thiamine"; however, in 1969 the American Institute of Nutrition formally adopted the spelling without the "e" and this preferred spelling has been used since that time in most scientific writings.

See Vitamin B$_1$

THIRST is the conscious desire for water. It is the way that we maintain the correct level of water in the body for normal functioning. It isn't always a reliable indicator of need, however, especially in older individuals. The sensation of thirst is caused by nerves in the hypothalamus of the brain which monitors the concentration of sodium in the blood. When the concentration of sodium increases, the nerve cells transmit the sensation of thirst. It takes only a one percent change in the concentration of sodium in the blood to make a person feel thirsty.

See Water

TOCOPHEROL is a chemical name for vitamin E. There are alpha, beta and gamma forms of this nutrient.

See Vitamin E

TOFU is soybean cheese or bean curd.

See Soybeans, Bean curd

TOFUTTI is a soybean-based, nondairy alternative to ice cream.

See Soybeans

TOTAL PARENTERAL NUTRITION, *see* TPN

TOXINS are poisons. Some are produced by bacteria and others are substances naturally occurring in food which can be harmful when eaten in large amounts. Natural toxins in foods have caused serious illness and death throughout history. Potato poisoning was common in areas of the world where potatoes were eaten in large amounts at times of food shortages. Even today a

Natural Toxins in Food

Substance	Food Source	Toxic Effect	Comments
Goitrogens	cabbage, kale, brussels sprouts, cauliflower, broccoli, turnips, watercress, radish	induce goiter by interfering with the body's use of iodine	Cooking these vegetables inactivates goitrogenic activity.
Estrogens	soybeans, soybean sprouts, alfalfa, carrots, wheat, rice, oats, barley, potatoes, apples, cherries, cottonseed oil, safflower oil, wheat germ oil, olive oil	responsible for cases of livestock infertility	Quantity of estrogen present is too low to cause any effect in the body.
Vasoactive amines tyramine dopamine norepinephrine serotonin histamine	plantains, bananas, ripened cheese, avocados, soybeans, meat broth, liver, pineapple juice	elevation in blood pressure; migraine headaches	These amines are usually inactivated by an enzyme normally present in body; mood-elevating drugs can inhibit this enzyme.

Tyrpsin inhibitor	soybeans, lima beans, mung beans, peanuts, oats, buckwheat, barley, sweet potato, peas, corn, white potato	interferes with digestion and absorption of protein	Cooking destroys the inhibitor.
Solanin	potatoes (most potent), apples, eggplant	interferes with transmission of nerve impulses; poisoning	Not destroyed in cooking—found mainly in skins.
Alkaloidlike compounds and cyclopeptides	mushrooms	poisoning	Only a small number of mushroom species are poisonous; domestically cultivated mushrooms are free of toxic substances; never harvest mushrooms from an unknown source.
Cyanide	apricot pits or kernels, peach pits, kernel paste, cassava, cashew nuts, lima beans, kirsch liqueur	cyanide poisoning	The controversial cancer treatment Laetrile is made with apricot kernels.

Substance	Food Source	Toxic Effect	Comments
Glycyrrhizic acid	licorice	severe hypertension, water retention, enlarged heart	Daily eating of large amounts of licorice candy has caused some symptoms; not found in artifically flavored licorice.
Menthol	candy, gums, liqueurs, cigarettes, toothpaste, mouthwash	hives, heart fibrillation, psychosis	Severe symptoms have been reported due to addiction to mentholated cigarettes or peppermint candy.
Myristicin	nutmeg, mace, black pepper, carrots, parsley, celery, dill	headache, cramps, nausea, poisoning	Large amounts of nutmeg or mace result in symptoms similar to drunkenness and can be poisonous.
Aflatoxins	peanuts, peanut butter, other nuts, corn, wheat	liver damage; carcinogenic	Domestic peanuts and imported nuts are monitored for contamination.

256

Antivitamins avidin Thiaminase Citral	egg whites, blackberries, black currants, red beets, brussels sprouts, red cabbage, spinach, raw fish, orange peel, marmalade	Inactivates biotin inactivates thiamine (B_1) inhibits vitamin A	An antivitamin diminishes or destroys the effect of a vitamin in the body; avidin and some forms of thiaminase are destroyed by cooking.
Safrole	oil of sassafras	carcinogenic	Prohibited in our food supply since 1958.
Thujone	herbal teas containing sage, yarrow or wormwood, vermouth	poisoning, convulsions	Allergic reactions have occurred from chronic use of herbal teas with yarrow.
Psoralens	parsley, parsnips, figs, limes, caraway	photosensitizers resulting in unusual sensitivity to sun causing severe sunburn	Large portion destroyed in cooking.
Benzopyrene	charcoal-broiled meat, olive oil, smoked meats	carcinogenic	
Nitrates	beets, spinach, radishes, lettuce, drinking water	carcinogenic	

Substance	Food Source	Toxic Effect	Comments
Phenols	rhubarb, St. John's-wort, buckwheat, cashew, mangos, nutmeg, sassafras, honey, apples	poisoning	Plant poisonings are responsible for 4% of all accidental poisonings each year—most occur in small children
Oxalates	spinach, Swiss chard, beets, greens, rhubarb	inhibits absorption of calcium	Rhubarb leaves contain 3 to 4 times as much as stalk and can result in illness if eaten raw.
Phytate	cereals, nuts, dried peas and beans, wheat germ	inhibits absorption of calcium, zinc, iron, magnesium	High-fiber diets are rich in phytates.

258

few cases of mushroom poisoning are reported yearly to the National Center for Poison Control.

All the foods listed on pp. 254–58 are safe when eaten as part of a balanced and varied diet. Their potential risk is tiny but none the less present. Overenthusiastic or unskilled naturalists, food faddists or those who have bizarre diets may be at risk. Most of us are not.

TPN stands for total parenteral nutrition and refers to a method of feeding where all of the person's nutrient needs are provided by intravenous means. TPN is usually used when a person cannot be fed through the digestive tract because it is diseased or a part of it has been surgically removed. It can be used temporarily or permanently. The nutrients are passed into a large vein, usually the vena cava, near the heart. This procedure was begun in the 1950s. Today, it has reached such a degree of technological sophistication that patients can do the procedure themselves at home and continue to lead a normal and complete life, though traditional eating and digesting is not possible.

TREE EAR, also called mo-er, black tree fungus, cloud ear and wood ears, is an edible Chinese fungus believed to have anti-blood-clotting properties. Biochemists at George Washington University have identified the anticlotting substance in the fungus as adenosine, a chemical also found in garlic and onions. Adenosine interferes with the clumping of blood cells, which plays a crucial role in blood clot formation. Someday, this food may be an effective tool in the prevention of atherosclerosis.

TRIGLYCERIDES are a type of fat made up of three fatty acids attached to a glycerol molecule. Almost all the fats and oils found in food and the fat in our bodies is in the form of triglycerides.

See Hypertriglyceridemia, Sucrose polyester

TRYPTOPHAN is an amino acid found in high amounts in animal foods. It provides the building blocks to make the neurotransmitter serotonin. Neurotransmitters are chemical substances that help transmit nerve impulses. In controlled experiments, people who reported difficulty sleeping were successfully treated when they took 5 to 10 gm of tryptophan. This is a very high dose when compared to the amount of tryptophan eaten in food, therefore self-medication with tryptophan for sleep disturbances should be approached with caution.

TYRAMINE is an amino acid found in large amounts in aged cheese (Cheddar, Gruyere, Stilton, Brie, Emmantaler), certain wines and other foods. A group of antidepressant drugs called "monoamine oxidase inhibitors" (MAOI's) can react very dramatically with tyramine-containing foods and cause a high blood pressure crisis. Small amounts of tyramine can cause a response, while larger amounts are dangerous. Parnate, Eutonyl and Nardil are MAOI's.

FOOD HIGH IN TYRAMINE

Cheese:
Blue
Brie
Cheddar
Emmantaler
Gruyere
Mozzarella
Roquefort
Stilton
Other foods:
Avocados
Bananas
Beer

Bologna
Canned figs
Cheese-containing foods
   (like casseroles)
Chianti wine
Chocolate
Dates
Fava beans
Liver
Meat extracts (like Marmite
   and Bovril)
Meat tenderizers
Nuts
Papaya
Patés
Pickled and kippered
   herring
Pepperoni
Raisins
Salami
Sausage
Sherry
Soups (canned and
   instant)
Sour cream
Soy sauce
Vanilla
Yeast or yeast
   extracts
Yogurt

U

ULCERS are open sores or erosions of the surface lining of the digestive tract. They are roughly similar to canker sores in the mouth. Ulcers can occur in any part of the digestive tract but are most common in the upper part of the small intestine, the duodendum (called duodenal ulcers) and in the stomach (called gastric ulcers). Both types may be referred to as peptic ulcers. It's estimated that about 10 percent of the population has an ulcer at some point and the incidence of recurrence is high. There are numerous explanations for the cause—heredity, emotional stress, drug irritation, poor nutrition, lack of rest. The idea that stomach acid causes ulcers is false. Once an ulcer is formed, stomach acid may irritate and worsen the condition but the acid did not cause it.

Gone are the days of drinking heavy cream to "soothe" the ulcer, eating pureed fruits and vegetables and avoiding gassy foods. Milk is not a good buffer and may stimulate acid secretion, causing more harm than good. A moderate amount of fiber is not irritating and helps avoid constipation. Each person reacts differently to gassy foods; what causes discomfort for one will not for another. Even eating frequent meals has been challenged but is usually still recommended. Today there is no clear-cut ulcer diet. Persons are encouraged to eat normally and simply avoid any food that causes them pain or discomfort.

UNDERNOURISHED refers to taking in too little food (Calories and nutrients) to meet the needs of the body. If the condition is chronic, weight loss and then malnutrition will result.

UNDERWEIGHT is a word with various meanings. Some believe it just means desired slimness; to others it can be equal to malnutrition. Technically the term means a body weight that is low for the person's age, height and sex. Being 10 percent below ideal weight is usually considered underweight. A person who is underweight may lack body reserves of fat, muscle and nutrients which can affect their health.

In the early 1900s, underweight people were charged higher life insurance premiums because they were more likely to get tuberculosis. Today the risk of getting tuberculosis is rare and overweight people often pay higher premiums. Chronic low weight, however, can cause such health problems as:

Irregular menstrual periods
Retarded growth in infants and children
Increased risk for infection
Lack of energy and sexual drive
Lowered resistance to stress (both physical and mental)
Slow healing
Greater tendency to be irritable, depressed, nervous, restless or sleepless
Weak muscles

U.S. Recommended Daily Allowances (U.S. RDA's)

Nutrients which must be declared on the label:*	Infants: birth to 12 months (tentative)	Children under 4 years of age	Adults and children 4 or more years of age	Pregnant or lactating women
Protein (g), PER** ≥ casein	20	45	45	45
Protein (g), PER < casein	28	65	65	65
Vitamin A (IU)	1,500	2,500	5,000	8,000
Vitamin C (Ascorbic acid) (mg)	35	45	60	60
Thiamin (vitamin B_1) (mg)	0.5	0.7	1.5	1.7
Riboflavin (vitamin B_2) (mg)	0.6	0.8	1.7	2
Niacin (mg)	8	9	20	20
Calcium (g)	0.6	0.8	1.0	1.3
Iron (mg)	15	10	18	18

Nutrients which may be declared or the label:				
Vitamin D (IU)	400	400	400	400
Vitamin E (IU)	5	10	30	30
Vitamin B$_6$ (mg)	0.4	0.7	2	2.5
Folic acid (folacin) (mg)	0.1	0.2	0.4	0.8
Vitamin B$_{12}$ (ug)	2	3	6	8
Phosphorus (g)	0.5	0.8	1	1.3
Iodine (ug)	45	70	150	150
Magnesium (mg)	70	200	400	400
Zinc (mg)	5	8	15	15
Copper (mg)	0.6	1	2	2
Biotin (mg)	0.05	0.15	0.3	0.3
Pantothenic acid (mg)	3	5	10	10

*whenever nutrition labeling is required
**Protein Efficiency Rating

URIC ACID, *see* Gout

U.S. RECOMMENDED DAILY ALLOWANCES (U.S. RDA) are standards used for nutrition labeling. They are based on the Recommended Dietary Allowances (RDA) but are a simplification that is more appropriate for a food label. They have a single value for each nutrient instead of the range of values for different ages and sexes in the RDA. In most cases the value used is the highest recommendation for that nutrient, excepting pregnant and breast-feeding women. The value for protein is 45 gm if a product contains good quality protein (animal sources) and 65 gm if the protein is of lesser quality (vegetable sources). The minerals calcium and phosphorus are exceptions as their level is set at 1.0 gm for each. Recommended levels for other nutrients—which were not included in the RDA at the time nutrition labeling was established—have been determined individually.

On the label the nutrient composition of the food is given as a percent of the U.S. RDA.

U.S. RDA standards are listed on pages 264–65.

See Nutrition labeling

V

VEGETABLE OILS are enclosed in the seeds and fruits of plants. Pressure must be applied to break the plant tissue to release the oil. Olive, mustard seed, palm and coconut oils were probably among the first oils used by man.

Most vegetable oils are high in polyunsaturated fatty acids and are recommended for use instead of saturated (animal) fats. Some oils are classified as monounsaturated—olive, peanut, rapeseed. Newer research shows they may be beneficial for certain types of heart disease. Palm oil and coconut oil are more like saturated (animal) fat than any other vegetable oil. For this reason they should be used in limited amounts. They are often found in nondairy creamers and whipped toppings and frozen desserts.

Following is a list of commonly used vegetable oils and their plant sources.

OIL	SOURCE
Coconut	nut of the coconut palm tree
Corn	corn grain
Cottonseed	seed of the cotton plant
Nut	a variety of nuts may be used such as walnut or hazelnut
Olive	olives
Palm	oil palm tree
Peanut	peanut, which is a member of the pea family, not a nut
Rapeseed	rape plant, a type of mustard plant
Safflower	safflower, a relative of the thistle
Sesame	sesame seeds
Sorghum	sorghum grain

VEGETABLES are plants or parts of plants that we eat as food. They contribute some calories, vitamins, minerals, fiber and water to the diet. Interestingly, many of the vegetables commonly eaten in the United States did not originate on this continent. Following is a list of common vegetables and their place of origin.

VEGETABLE	PLACE OF ORIGIN
Artichoke	Mediterranean region
Asparagus	Mediterranean region
Bean, snap	Mexico and Peru
Bean, lima	Peru
Beet	Europe and Asia
Broccoli	Europe
Brussels sprouts	Belgium
Cabbage	Europe
Carrot	Central Asia
Cauliflower	Asia
Celery	France or Italy
Corn	Mexico and South America
Cucumber	Southeast Asia
Eggplant	India
Garlic	Central Asia

Vegetable	Place of Origin
Lettuce	Egypt
Okra	Ethiopia
Olive	Greece
Onion	Central Asia
Pepper, green	Central and South America
Potato	South America
Radish	Egypt
Soybean	China
Squash	Mexico and Central America
Sweet potato	Mexico, Central America, South America
Tomato	South America
Turnip	Europe

VEGETARIANS may be defined, in the strictest sense, as those who eat only foods of plant origin—no meat, fish, poultry, eggs, milk or cheese. This practice varies considerably. Those who do not eat animal products are called *vegans*. *Lactovegetarians* supplement plant foods with dairy products—milk, yogurt, cheese, ice cream, etc. *Lacto-ovovegetarians* eat plant foods, dairy foods and eggs. Others are less traditional in their eating practices and may eat poultry and/or fish, insist on eating only organically grown produce or limit their intake in other individualized ways. Today, vegetarian practices may conform to a person's religious, ecological or philosophical ideas. These wide differences can lead to problems in obtaining adequate nutrition.

Vegetarians have to be careful to get enough energy (Calories), protein, calcium, iron, vitamin D and vitamin B_{12}. Many of these nutrients are predominantly found in foods of animal origin. Vegetarians who eat some animal foods, like milk, eggs or fish, will get all the nutrients they need. Vegans need to plan their diet more carefully. Infants and children are particularly vulnerable to nutrient shortages on a strict vegan diet.

Most authorities advise a lacto-ovo or lactovegetarian diet for the growing child. The vegetarian four food groups (see below) can be used as a guide to daily meal planning.

With careful planning, vegetarian eating can be quite healthy and may bring with it some long-range benefits. It has been estimated that becoming and remaining a vegetarian may add as much as ten years to your expected life span by reducing the risk of obesity, diabetes, heart disease, cancer and osteoporosis.

Vegetarians are leaner than most meat eaters by an average of ten to twenty pounds. Even those who begin this way of eating later in life report a weight loss. Switching from a reliance on animal protein to a diet high in legumes (dried peas and beans), grains and other plant foods lowers cholesterol and total fat in the diet. Even lacto-ovovegetarians have lower serum cholesterols and lowered risk for heart disease. Strong evidence linking vegetarianism and a lessened risk of cancer has not yet been found. In the meantime, population trends point to a smaller number of cancers among vegetarians, suggesting more study may uncover a link. Osteoporosis begins to be evident in meat eaters after age 40. Vegetarians have 50 percent less bone thinning at age 60 and have consistently thicker and stronger bones up to the age of 89.

See Protein complementation, Zen macrobiotics

Vegetarian Four Food Groups

Milk (Use low-fat or 2% milk and milk products)

   2 or more servings daily

   1 serving   = 1 cup milk

   1 cup milk = 1½ ounces cheese

               = 2 cups cottage cheese

               = 1 cup pudding

               = 1 cup custard

1 cup milk = 1 cup yogurt
          = 1½ cups ice cream
          = 1 cup cooked collard greens
          = 1½ cups cooked kale, mustard greens,
             dandelion greens
          = 2 cups okra
          = 1⅓ cups cooked bok choy
          = 2½ ounces sardines

Legumes*, Nuts, Seeds and Eggs (Meat Substitutes)
  2 servings daily
  1 serving = 1 cup legumes
            = ¼ cup peanut butter
            = 6 ounces tofu (soybean curd)
            = 2 eggs
            = 2 slices cheese
            = ½ cup cottage cheese
            = 1½ ounces or 3 tablespoons nuts or seeds

Fruits and Vegetables
  4 or more servings daily. A food rich in vitamin C is
recommended daily
  1 serving = 1 medium whole fruit or vegetable (raw
               or cooked)
            = ½ cup cooked vegetable or fruit
            = ½ large fruit (i.e., grapefruit)
            = 2 to 3 small fruits (i.e., plum)
            = ½ cup (4 ounces) juice
            = 2 tablespoons dried fruit
            = 1 cup raw bulky or leaf vegetable (i.e.,
               spinach or bean sprouts)

Grains—Bread, Cereal, Pasta, Rice
  6 or more servings daily
  1 serving = 1 slice of bread
            = 1 cup cold cereal
            = ½ cup cooked cereal

---

*Dried peas, beans and peanuts

1 serving = ¼ to ⅓ cup granola-type cereal
= 1 tablespoon wheat germ
= ¾ cup brown rice
= ¾ cup pasta or noodles
= 1 biscuit, muffin, or pancake
= 1 slice nut or fruit bread
= 4 crackers
= 1 tablespoon nutritional yeast

VINEGAR The name *vinaigre* is French for sour wine. The bacteria *acetobactel* sours the wine, dissipates the alcohol and leaves a mixture of acetic acid and water. Historically vinegar was a by-product of wine makers and brewers. Today it is made from rice and other grains, apples, as well as wine. Vinegar is described in the Old Testament. It is used to prepare salad dressing and pickles and was once used by Cleopatra to dissolve a pearl to make what might have been the world's most expensive cocktail. Apple cider vinegar has been recommended as a folk treatment for arthritis. There is no scientific basis for this use.

VITAMIN A is needed in the body for the health of the eyes, mucous membranes and skin, and to ensure the growth of bones and teeth. About half of your daily requirement comes from fruits and vegetables and half comes from milk, cheese, eggs and meats. Those vegetables with the highest vitamin A are brightly colored—green, yellow-orange, and red. Pale yellow foods like corn or pineapple and white foods like onions and potatoes have little or no vitamin A. In plants, vitamin A is found as carotene, which is converted in your body to the active form of vitamin A.

Up to a year's supply of vitamin A is stored in the liver so it is hard to become deficient; it is more likely that a person could take too much. Adults should not take more than six times the RDA or 30,000 IU as a regular daily supplement; children and pregnant women should not take more than 10,000 IU daily. Taking large doses for prolonged periods can cause blurred vision, headaches, rashes, loss of appetite, hair loss, joint pain, liver damage and abnormal bone growth.

See Beta carotene, Hypervitaminosis, Megadoses, Retinol, Vitamins

Sources of Vitamin A

Food	Amount	IU
Liver, beef, fried	3 ounces	45,420
Mango	1 medium	11,000
Sweet potato, baked	1 medium	9,230
Pumpkin, canned	½ cup	8,000
Carrot, raw	1 medium	7,900
Spinach, cooked	½ cup	7,290
Carrots, diced, cooked	½ cup	7,110
Papaya	1 medium	5,300
Collards, cooked	½ cup	5,130
Product 19, Kellogg's	1 cup	5,000
Most, Kellogg's	1 cup	5,000
Winter squash, cooked	½ cup	4,900
Swiss chard, cooked	½ cup	4,700
Persimmon	1 medium	4,600
Broccoli, cooked	1 stalk	4,500
Pepper, red, raw	1 medium	3,300
Taco Bell Burrito Supreme	1	3,462
Taco Bell Tostado	1	3,152
Watermelon balls	1 cup	2,500
Cantaloupe	⅛	2,310
Nectarine	1 medium	2,300
All Bran	⅔ cup	1,563

Food	Amount	IU
Peach	1 medium	1,330
Wendy's Chili	1 cup	1,188
Tomato, raw	1 medium	1,100
Apricot	1 medium	960
Tomato juice	½ cup	950
Endive, raw	1 cup	800
Escarole, raw	1 cup	800
McDonald's Quarter Pounder with Cheese	1	660
Grapefruit, pink	½	630
Jack in the Box Super Taco	1	599
Egg	1	590
Asparagus, cooked	4 spears	540
Milk, skim	1 cup	500
Lettuce	¼ head	450
Peas, cooked	½ cup	430
Cucumber, raw, unpeeled	1 small	420
Summer squash, diced	½ cup	410
Ice cream	½ cup	390
Cheddar cheese	1 ounce	370
Romaine, raw	1 leaf	360
American cheese	1 ounce	350
Yellow corn,* canned	½ cup	345
Yogurt, whole milk	1 cup	340
Green beans, cooked	½ cup	340
Pepper, green, raw	1 medium	310
Milk	1 cup	300
Orange, navel	1 medium	280
Orange juice	½ cup	250
Lima beans, cooked	½ cup	240
Cottage cheese, creamed	½ cup	210
Yogurt, low-fat	1 cup	170
Margarine	1 teaspoon	155

---

*White corn contains little vitamin A.

Food	Amount	IU
Butter	1 teaspoon	155
Wax beans, canned	½ cup	140
Pineapple juice, canned	½ cup	65
Cabbage, shredded	½ cup	45
Bartlett pear	1 medium	30
Lentils, cooked	½ cup	20

The RDA for vitamin A is:	5000 IU males
	4000 IU females
The U.S. RDA (labeling tool) for vitamin A is:	5000 IU

VITAMIN B₁ is also called thiamin. It is necessary in the body for the release of energy and to keep nerves healthy. Deficiencies of this vitamin will affect the digestive tract, nervous system and heart. The classic deficiency disease, beri-beri, results from an extreme thiamin deficiency. In the United States this is seen mostly in alcoholics. Vitamin B₁ is found in a wide variety of foods but only a few foods contain it in large amounts. Pork, sunflower seeds, cornflakes and peanuts are the richest sources. Enriched breads and cereals have added B₁.

See Beri-beri, Enrichment, Megadoses, Thiamin, Vitamins

Sources of Thiamin (B₁)

Food	Amount	Milligrams
Product 19, Kellogg's	1 cup	1.5
Brewer's yeast	1 tablespoon	1.2
Pork	3 ounces	.91
Jack in the Box Pancakes	1 serving	.63
Dairy Queen Banana Split	1	.60
Morningstar Farms sausages	3	.60

Food	Amount	Milligrams
Arby's Super Roast Beef Sandwich	1 sandwich	.53
Special K, Kellogg's	1 cup	.53
Wendy's Double Hamburger with cheese	1	.49
Noodles, cooked	1 cup	.45
McDonald's Big Mac	1	.39
Kix, General Mills	1½ cups	.38
Cocoa Krispies	1 cup	.38
Taco Bell Combination Burrito	1	.34
Whole-wheat flour	½ cup	.33
Kentucky Fried Chicken Extra Crispy (drumstick and thigh)	1	.32
Carnation Breakfast Bar	1	.30
Instant Oatmeal, Quaker	1 envelope	.30
Pinto beans, cooked	½ cup	.26
Ham	3 ounces	.25
Oysters	¾ cup	.25
Orange	1 large	.24
Liver, beef	3 ounces	.23
Avocado	½ medium	.23
Peas	½ cup	.22
Wheat germ	2 tablespoons	.22
Black beans	½ cup	.18
Lima beans	½ cup	.16
Collard greens	½ cup	.14
Navy beans, cookedf	½ cup	.14
Lamb, leg	3 ounces	.13
Spinach, cooked	½ cup	.13
Asparagus	½ cup	.12
Orange juice	½ cup	.11
Veal roast	3 ounces	.11
Milk, 2% fat	8 ounces	.10

Food	Amount	Milligrams
Spaghetti	½ cup	.10
Macaroni	½ cup	.10
Oatmeal, cooked	½ cup	.10
Skim milk	8 ounces	.09
Potato	1 small	.08
Bran flakes	½ cup	.07
Whole milk	8 ounces	.07
Puffed rice	1 cup	.07
Tomatoes, cooked	½ cup	.06
Brussels sprouts	½ cup	.06
White bread	1 slice	.06
Whole-wheat bread	1 slice	.06
Broccoli	½ cup	.06
Egg	1	.05
Green beans	½ cup	.05
Chicken	3 ounces	.05

The RDA for thiamin is: 1.4 mg males
1.0 mg females

The U.S. RDA (labeling tool) for thiamin is: 1.5 mg

VITAMIN B$_2$ is also known as riboflavin. Milk is one of the richest sources of B$_2$, contributing about 50 percent of our daily need. Sunlight, however, can destroy B$_2$ so don't leave the milk container bathing in the morning sunlight on the breakfast table. Greens, breads and cereals are other good sources. Enriched breads and cereals have B$_2$ added. Vitamin B$_2$ is needed to use energy in the body and ensure healthy eyes, skin, lips and tongue.

See Enrichment, Megadoses, Vitamins

Sources of Riboflavin (B₂)

Food	Amount	Milligrams
Liver, beef	3 ounces	3.60
Most, Kellogg's	1 cup	1.7
Dairy Queen Malt, regular	1	.60
Milk, 2% fat	8 ounces	.52
Skim milk	8 ounces	.44
Yogurt, low-fat	8 ounces	.44
McDonald's Egg McMuffin	1	.44
Crispix, Kellogg's	¾ cup	.43
Arby's Beef and Cheese	1 sandwich	.43
Milk, regular	8 ounces	.41
Yogurt, whole milk	8 ounces	.39
Taco Bell Beef Burrito	1	.39
Wendy's Single Hamburger	1	.36
Instant Cream of Wheat	1 envelope	.34
Brewer's yeast	1 tablespoon	.34
Chipped beef	3 ounces	.30
Camembert cheese	1⅓-oz. wedge	.29
Broccoli, cooked	¾ cup	.27
Squash, butternut, baked	1 cup	.27
Veal, roast	3 ounces	.26
Lamb	3 ounces	.23
Avocado	½ medium	.23
Roast beef, lean	3 ounces	.19
Collard greens, cooked	½ cup	.19
Hamburger, cooked	3 ounces	.18
Sardines	3 ounces	.17
Ham	3 ounces	.16
Chicken	3 ounces	.16
Egg	1	.15
Okra, cooked	½ cup	.15
Cottage cheese, creamed	¼ cup	.15
Mushrooms	½ cup	.14
Asparagus, cooked	½ cup	.13
Cheddar cheese	1 ounce	.13
Spinach, cooked	½ cup	.13

Food	Amount	Milligrams
Broccoli, cooked	½ cup	.12
Spaghetti, cooked	1 cup	.12
Beet greens, cooked	½ cup	.11
Tuna, canned	3 ounces	.10
Wheat germ	2 tablespoons	.10
Lima beans, cooked	½ cup	.09
Peas, cooked	½ cup	.09
Corn muffin	1	.08
Carnation Instant Breakfast	1 envelope	.07
Pancake	1	.06
White bread	1 slice	.05
Cauliflower, cooked	½ cup	.05
Orange	1 medium	.05

The RDA for riboflavin is: 1.6 mg males
1.2 mg females

The U.S. RDA (labeling tool) for riboflavin is: 1.7 mg

VITAMIN B_6 is also known as pyridoxine. B_6 is found in meats, milk, breads and cereal. High heat can destroy it. Its major function is to release energy in the body and to help with the formation of new red blood cells. B_6 is used to relieve nausea and vomiting in early pregnancy and lozenges containing B_6 have been used to prevent dental cavities. Large doses can be dangerous, causing muscle incoordination and nerve damage. It has been suggested as a treatment for premenstrual syndrome (PMS) but no effective proof has been shown. In some cases the Chinese Restaurant Syndrome is caused by a deficiency of vitamin B_6, aggravated by a large dose of MSG (monosodium glutamate).

See Hypervitaminosis, Megadoses, MSG, Premenstrual syndrome, Vitamins

Sources of Vitamin B₆ (Pyridoxine)

Food	Amount	Milligrams
Most, Kellogg's	1 cup	2.0
Tuna, canned	3½ ounces	.90
Liver	3 ounces	.84
Chicken	3½ ounces	.70
Corn Flakes, Kellogg's	1 cup	.70
Banana	1 medium	.61
Kix, General Mills	1½ cups	.50
Avocado	½ medium	.46
Pork	3 ounces	.45
Beef	3 ounces	.44
Halibut	3 ounces	.43
Brussels sprouts, cooked	4 large	.40
Carnation Instant Breakfast	1 envelope	.40
Egg yolk	1	.30
Corn, canned	½ cup	.30
Sunflower seeds	2 tablespoons	.22
Brewer's yeast	1 tablespoon	.20
Cottage cheese, creamed	½ cup	.20
Asparagus, cooked	½ cup	.20
Summer squash, cooked	½ cup	.20
Wheat germ	2 tablespoons	.15
Frankfurter	1	.14
Lima beans, cooked	½ cup	.12
Cantaloupe	¼ melon	.12
Peanut butter	2 tablespoons	.11
Tomato	1 medium	.10
Yogurt	8 ounces	.10
Spoon Size Shredded Wheat	1 cup	.10
Peanuts	2 tablespoons	.10

The RDA for vitamin B₆ is: 2.2 mg males
                                                      2.0 mg females

The U.S. RDA (labeling tool) for vitamin B₆ is: 2.0 mg

VITAMIN B$_{12}$ is also called cobalamin. Your daily need for B$_{12}$, 3 micrograms, weighs about as much as the ink used to make the period at the end of this sentence. It is unique in the B vitamin family in that it is found almost exclusively in animal foods. The vitamin is sensitive to heat and can be destroyed by long cooking. Strict vegetarians could be short of this vitamin unless they drink B$_{12}$ fortified soy milk or take a supplement. This vitamin is needed for the release of energy and for the normal functioning of all cells but particularly those of the bone marrow, nervous system and digestive tract. A deficiency of B$_{12}$ or a lack of the intrinsic factor, a protein substance necessary for the absorption of B$_{12}$, can lead to pernicious anemia. *Pernicious* means fatal and this type of anemia was just that until it was discovered in the 1920s that feeding liver and liver extract cured the problem. Today, this form of anemia is treated by injections of B$_{12}$.

See Anemia, Megadoses, Vitamins

Sources of Vitamin B$_{12}$

Food	Amount	Micrograms
Liver, beef	3½ ounces	80.0
Liver, chicken	3½ ounces	24.1
Clams, canned	½ cup	20.0
Oysters, raw	3½ ounces	18.0
Liverwurst	2 slices	9.2
Crabmeat, canned	3½ ounces	8.5
Sardines	3½ ounces	8.3
Salmon, canned	3½ ounces	7.5
Product 19, Kellogg's	1 cup	6.0
Tuna fish	3½ ounces	3.0
Morningstar Farms sausages	3	2.4
Beefsteak	3 ounces	2.2
Hamburger	3 ounces	1.8
Veal, lean	3½ ounces	1.8

Food	Amount	Micrograms
Haddock	3½ ounces	1.7
Lamb	3½ ounces	1.6
Kix, Kellogg's	1½ cups	1.5
Yogurt	8 ounces	1.3
Flounder	3½ ounces	1.2
Milk	1 cup	1.0
Ham	3½ ounces	.8
Cottage cheese	½ cup	.7
Egg	1	.6
Carnation Breakfast Bar	1	.6
Buttermilk	8 ounces	.5
Swiss cheese*	1 ounce	.5
Bleu cheese*	1 ounce	.4
Camembert cheese*	1 ounce	.4
Cheddar cheese*	1 ounce	.3

The RDA for vitamin B_{12} is: 3 mcg

The U.S. RDA (labeling tool) for vitamin B_{12} is: 6 mcg

*As cheese ripens, the amount of B vitamins increases.

VITAMIN B_{15} is also called pangamate and pangamic acid. It is not a vitamin because it is not needed to prevent a deficiency disease, and is classified as a food additive by the Food and Drug Administration. It was named in the early 1950s by E. T. Krebs, who isolated the substance from apricot pits; he used it to treat cancer. His treatment was unsuccessful and sometimes dangerous.

Supporters claim B_{15} increases oxygen uptake by blood and tissues resulting in more energy and lowered blood cholesterol. It is promoted as a treatment for cardiovascular disease including arteriosclerosis, shortness of breath, chest pain; for athletes to increase physical endurance; for liver disease; and for skin disorders and tumors. Most of these treatments were developed in the United Soviet Socialist Republic where pangamic acid is manufactured and widely distributed. The use of this substance is controversial. More research is needed to clarify its role in the human body.

Pangamic acid is found in foods along with the B vitamin family. Sunflower seeds, pumpkin seeds, rice, yeast and liver are food sources.

At the current time over fifty companies make B_{15}, but none of them follows Krebs's original formula because no one knows what that formula was. When scientists analyzed different brands of B_{15}, they found each brand was different. One was pure lactose (milk sugar); another PABA (part of the B vitamin folic acid); and others contained known cancer-causing substances. The only people who benefit from B_{15} are those who sell it.

See Laetrile, Vitamin B_{17}

VITAMIN B_{17} is another name for the questionable anticancer drug Laetrile. The Food and Drug Administration has banned the sale of B_{17} supplements in the United States.

See Laetrile

VITAMIN C is also known as ascorbic acid. It performs a variety of important functions: helping the cells to cement together; aiding in the formation of bones, teeth, cartilage, connective tissue and blood vessels; helping to make new red blood cells in the bone marrow; assisting in the absorption of other nutrients like iron; and possibly helping the body to resist infection.

Centuries ago, sailors on long ocean voyages often died of scurvy caused by a deficiency of vitamin C.

Today this is highly unlikely since it is found in many commonly eaten fruits and vegetables, the best known being orange juice. Today the concern is from excessive intakes of C. It is a popular vitamin and people frequently take it in large amounts. Daily doses up to 2,000 milligrams (2 grams) appear to cause little harm. Doses above this can result in serious side effects from diarrhea to distorting lab values on important diagnostic tests for diabetes, gout and cancer of the colon.

See Megadoses, Scurvy, Vitamins

Sources of Vitamin C

Food	Amount	Milligrams
Guava	1 medium	240
Papaya	1 medium	170
Red pepper	1 medium	150
Green pepper	1 medium	94
Collard greens, cooked	½ cup	70
Orange	1 medium	66
Brussels sprouts	½ cup	63
Orange juice, fresh	½ cup	62
Orange juice, frozen	½ cup	60
Product 19, Kellogg's	1 cup	60
Grape juice, Seneca, frozen	6 ounces	60
Cranapple, Ocean Spray	6 ounces	60
Lipton Iced Tea, ready to drink	8 ounces	60
Most, Kellogg's	1 cup	60
Grapefruit	½	54
Broccoli	½ cup	53
Orange juice, canned	½ cup	50
Green pepper	½	47
Cantaloupe	¼	45
Strawberries	½ cup	44
Cauliflower	½ cup	33

Food	Amount	Milligrams
Potato, baked	1 medium	31
Watermelon	1 slice	30
Tomato, cooked	½ cup	29
Persimmon	1 medium	29
Tomato	1 medium	28
Spinach, raw	1 cup	28
Tangerine	1 medium	27
Carnation Breakfast Bar, chocolate chip	1 bar	27
Carnation Instant Breakfast, chocolate	1 envelope	27
Pineapple, diced	1 cup	26
Sweet potato, baked	1 medium	25
Spinach, cooked	½ cup	25
Cabbage, cooked	½ cup	24
Liver, beef	3 ounces	23
Potato, boiled	1 medium	22
Passionfruit	1 medium	20
Plantain	½ medium	20
Tomato juice	½ cup	19
Lemonade	1 cup	17
Peas, cooked	½ cup	16
Lima beans, cooked	½ cup	15
Tomato soup	1 cup	15
Corn Flakes, Kellogg's	1 cup	15
Taco Bell Bean Burrito	1	15
Sapodilla	1 medium	15
McDonald's Regular Fries	1 serving	13
Banana	1 medium	12
Cocoa Krispies, Kellogg's	1 cup	11
Bean sprouts, mung	½ cup	10
Potato, instant mashed	½ cup	6
Potato chips	10	3

The RDA for vitamin C is: 60 mg

The U.S. RDA (labeling tool) for vitamin C is: 60 mg

VITAMIN D is often called the sunshine vitamin because a substance just under the skin can be converted to vitamin D when the skin is exposed to ultraviolet light from the sun. Clothing, time indoors, shortened winter days and skin color can affect how much vitamin D the body makes. Sunshine cannot be relied on to supply all our need; vitamin D fortified milk is the major source. Fortification of milk began as a response to rickets, a bone deforming disease of infants and children caused by a lack of vitamin D. Though rickets is rare today, occasionally a breast-fed baby or one given a nondairy, nonfortified milk substitute will become deficient.

Overdoses of vitamin D are far more likely. As little as 2,000 IU—only five times the recommended daily requirement—has been toxic to children.

See Hypervitaminosis, Megadoses, Vitamins

Sources of Vitamin D

Food	Amount	IU
Product 19, Kellogg's	1 cup	200
Most, Kellogg's	1 cup	200
Dairy Queen Malt	large	140
Ovaltine	1 cup	139
Milk, fortified	1 cup	100
Skim milk, fortified	1 cup	100
Jack in the Box		
Breakfast Jack sandwich	1	51
McDonald's Egg McMuffin	1	46
Liver, beef, cooked	2½ ounces	46
Liver, pork, cooked	2½ ounces	46
McDonald's Chocolate Shake	1	44
Special K, Kellogg's	1 cup	40
Crispix, Kellogg's	¾ cup	40
Kix, General Mills	1½ cups	40
ET Cereal, General Mills	1 cup	40

Food	Amount	IU
Milk Break, Milk Bar	1	40
McDonald's Big Mac	1	33
Egg	1 medium	27
Eggnog	½ cup	21
Chicken liver, cooked	2½ ounces	20
Liver, calves', cooked	2½ ounces	12
Butter	1 teaspoon	5
Cream, light	2 tablespoons	4
Meat loaf (beef and pork)	2½ ounces	2

The RDA for vitamin D is: 200 IU for adults

The U.S. RDA (labeling tool) for vitamin D is: 400 IU

VITAMIN E has the reputation of being able to enhance sexual potency. Unfortunately, this will only work on rats and not on humans. In the rat, a diet deficient in vitamin E leads to sterility; that's the beginning of this nutrition myth.

Sixty percent of the vitamin E in the diet comes from vegetable oils: sunflower, wheat germ, cottonseed, walnut, corn and sesame seed oils are very rich sources. Ten percent of our vitamin E comes from fruits and vegetables. Vitamin E can be broken down when frozen and it can be removed in some food processing, like refining of breads and cereals. Oils high in vitamin E should be stored in amber glass bottles in the refrigerator. Light and heat will speed up their spoilage and destroy their vitamin E content.

Chemical substances with vitamin E activity, i.e. the ability to act as coenzymes in metabolic reactions that require Vitamin E, are referred to as tocopherols. The precise role of these substances is unclear but they seem to protect other body compounds from attack by oxygen. They act as antioxidants both in the body and in food processing where they function as additives to ensure freshness. A deficiency of vitamin E is highly unlikely, as is an overdose. However, some unpleasant side effects have been reported from excessive intake.

See Megadoses, Tocopherols, Vitamins

Sources of Vitamin E

Food	Amount	IU
Total	1 cup	30.0
Most, Kellogg's	1 cup	30.0
Wheat germ oil	1 tablespoon	28.3
Walnut oil	1 tablespoon	13.1
Sunflower oil	1 tablespoon	10.3
Sweet potato	1 medium	9.7
Cottonseed oil	1 tablespoon	8.9
Safflower oil	1 tablespoon	8.5
Walnuts	11 halves	4.6
Asparagus	5–6 spears	3.7
Corn oil	1 tablespoon	3.6
Sunflower seeds	2 tablespoons	3.5
Soybean oil	1 tablespoon	3.4
Almonds	7 nuts	3.0
Hazelnuts	5 nuts	2.4
Brussels sprouts	3 large	2.3
Broccoli	1 cup	2.2
Wheat germ	2 tablespoons	2.1
Apple	1 medium	1.8
Beans, dry	½ cup	1.6
Corn	1 ear	1.5
Whole-wheat flour	⅓ cup	1.5
Parsnip	½ large	1.5
Brazil nuts	4 nuts	1.4
Peanuts	1 tablespoon	1.4
Pear	1 medium	1.2
Brown rice, uncooked	⅓ cup	1.1

Food	Amount	IU
Banana	1 medium	.7
Carrot	1 medium	.6
Egg	1 large	.6
Grapefruit	½ medium	.6
Plum	1 large	.6
Butter	1 tablespoon	.5
Tomato	1 medium	.5
Raspberries	½ cup	.4
Cornmeal, uncooked	¼ cup	.4
Oatmeal, uncooked	¼ cup	.4
Orange	1 medium	.4
Onions	1 medium	.3
Strawberries	½ cup	.3
Milk, regular	1 cup	.3
Spaghetti, uncooked	2 ounces	.2
Cherries	10	.2
White rice, uncooked	¼ cup	.1
White flour	¼ cup	.1
Whole-wheat bread	1 slice	.1

The RDA for vitamin E is: 10 IU for males
8 IU for females

The U.S. RDA (labeling tool) for vitamin E is: 30 IU

VITAMIN K is necessary for normal blood clotting. Daily need is small and can easily be met since many foods contain vitamin K. In addition, the "friendly" bacteria in the digestive tract produce a small but continuous supply. Deficiencies are rare but toxicity can occur if large doses of the synthetic form, *menadione*, are taken.

See Megadoses, Vitamins

Sources of Vitamin K*

Food	Amount	Micrograms
Turnip greens, cooked	⅔ cup	650
Lettuce	¼ head	129
Cabbage, cooked	⅔ cup	125
Liver, beef	3 ounces	110
Broccoli, cooked	½ cup	100
Spinach, cooked	½ cup	80
Asparagus, cooked	⅔ cup	57
Liver, pork	3 ounces	30
Peas, cooked	⅔ cup	19
Ham	3 ounces	18
Green beans, cooked	¾ cup	14
Cheese	1 ounce	14
Egg	1	11
Ground beef, raw	4 ounces	10.5
Milk	1 cup	10
Liver, chicken	3 ounces	8
Peach	1 medium	8
Butter	1 tablespoon	6
Tomato	1 small	5
Banana	1 medium	3
Applesauce	⅓ cup	2
Corn oil	1 tablespoon	2
Bread	1 slice	1

The RDA for vitamin K is: 70–140 mcg

There is no nutrition labeling recommendation for vitamin K.

---

*This nutrient is not found in the main table of the RDA because there is less information known about it; therefore a range of estimated safe and adequate daily dietary intake is suggested rather than a specific recommendation.

VITAMIN P is actually a bioflavonoid; it has not been considered a vitamin for over thirty-five years, since scientists discovered that it was not an essential nutrient for life. Rutin and hesperidin are part of this group. In nature, bioflavonoids are abundant in citrus fruit, blueberries, raspberries, watermelon, red cabbage, eggplant, tea, coffee, wine and beer. A typical diet averages 1,000 milligrams (1 gram) of bioflavonoids a day. Supplements are unnecessary.

See Bioflavonoids

VITAMINS are organic compounds needed in small amounts that are vital to life. The word is derived from *vita* meaning "life" and *amine* meaning "containing nitrogen." The major role that vitamins play in the body is to regulate the body processes that help fat, carbohydrate and protein to be digested, absorbed and metabolized.

Because vitamins are organic they can be destroyed, oxidized or changed in shape. This can be helpful since the body may alter the form of a vitamin to make it more useful in a given situation. The destructibility, however, can reduce the amount of vitamin in a food, if the food is improperly handled, stored or cooked.

Vitamins can be subdivided into two major categories: fat soluble (vitamins A, D, E and K) and water soluble (vitamin C and the B vitamin family). Each category of vitamins is absorbed, transported, stored and excreted in different ways by the body. Fat soluble vitamins are absorbed into the lymph system with other fat molecules; carried in the blood bound to protein molecules; and stored with fat in the body. This system can result in excessive storage of fat soluble vitamins when large doses are repeatedly taken for extended periods. The body does not have a method of easily excreting unneeded amounts of fat soluble vitamins, so toxicity (hypervitaminosis) may result.

Water soluble vitamins are absorbed across the intestinal wall directly into the blood where they travel freely around the body dissolved in the blood. As blood flows through the kidneys it detects high concentrations of substances in the blood and sets up the filtration system necessary to excrete the excess substances through the urine. Excess water soluble vitamins are removed from the body in this way, usually limiting their potential for toxicity. Due to the body's system for handling each type of vitamin, fat soluble vitamins may be taken in larger amounts less frequently since the extra can be stored for future use. Water soluble vitamins are needed more frequently (daily or every few days) and in smaller doses. The amount of water soluble vitamins held in the body may last for weeks or a few months. The storage of fat soluble vitamins could last for a number of years.

See Individual vitamin names, Megadoses, Multivitamin/mineral supplements

Fat Soluble	Water Soluble
A	C
D	B complex
E	B₁ (thiamin)
K	B₂ (riboflavin)
	Niacin
	Folic acid
	B₆
	B₁₂
	Pantothenic acid
	Biotin

Vitamins and Their Chemical Names

Vitamin	Chemical Name	Vitamin on Label
A	carotenoids, retinol	vitamin A palmitate beta carotene

Vitamin	Chemical Name	Vitamin on Label
B$_1$	thiamin	thiamine hydrochloride thiamine mononitrate
B$_2$	riboflavin	riboflavin-5 phosphate
Pantothenic acid (a B vitamin)	pantothenic acid	panthenol calcium pantothenate
Niacin (a B vitamin)	nicotinic acid nicotin amide	niacinamide
B$_6$	pyridoxine	pyridoxine hydrochloride (HCL)
B$_{12}$	cobalamin cyanocobalamin	cobalamin concentrate cyanocobalamin
Folic acid (a B vitamin)	folacin folic acid folate	folocin folic acid
Biotin (a B vitamin)	biotin	biotin
C	ascorbic acid	sodium ascorbate ascorbic acid
D	cholecalciferol	calciferol, ergocalciferol
E	tocopherol	alpha tocopherol mixed alpha tocopherols concentrate alpha tocopheryl acetate alpha tocopheryl acetate concentrate alpha tocopheryl acid succinate
K	naphthoquinone	phytonadione

Vitamin Functions and Sources

Vitamins	What They Do for You	Food Sources
A	Needed for growth and maintenance of eyes, skin, hair, teeth, bones and glands, and for resistance to infection; helps eyes adjust from light to darkness	Liver, eggs, butter, margarine, milk, dark green leafy and deep yellow vegetables and yellow fruit (spinach, broccoli, carrots, squash, sweet potatoes, apricots, mango)
B₁ (thiamin)	Helps release energy from food; needed for health of digestive and nervous systems and for maintenance of appetite	Whole-grain and enriched breads and cereals, liver, pork, wheat germ, dried peas and beans, nuts
B₂ (riboflavin)	Helps release energy fromn food; needed for health of skin, tongue, lips, eyes and nerves	Milk, yogurt, cheese, liver, meat, fish, poultry, eggs, enriched and whole-grain breads and cereals, deep green leafy vegetables
Niacin	Helps body cells produce energy; maintains health of skin, tongue, digestive system and nerves	Liver, peanuts, peanut butter, dried peas and beans, meat, poultry, fish, enriched and whole-grain breads and cereals, potatoes, milk, yeast

B$_6$ (pyridoxine)	Needed for use of carbohydrates, protein and fat, and for health of skin, lips, tongue, eyes and blood	Meat, poultry, fish, white and sweet potatoes, whole-grain breads and cereals, milk and yeast
B$_{12}$ (cyanocobalamin)	Needed for normal development of red blood cells and for normal function of nerves; helps build genetic material	Meat, poultry, fish, liver, cheese, eggs, milk
Folic acid	Needed for normal development of red blood cells and for normal use of protein; helps build genetic material	Liver, leafy green vegetables, meat, eggs, whole-grain breads and cereals
Pantothenic acid	Needed for use of carbohydrates, fat and protein, and for health of nerves	Eggs, whole-grain breads and cereals, liver, peanuts, dried peas and beans
Biotin	Needed for use of carbohydrates, fat and protein	Liver, meat, eggs and milk

Vitamins	What They Do for You	Food Sources
C	Needed for health of bones, teeth and blood vessels; helps hold body cells together, fights infection; aids iron absorption	Oranges, grapefruit, tangerines, lemons, limes, cantaloupe, strawberries, tomatoes, papaya, cabbage, broccoli, green peppers, white and sweet potatoes
D	Needed for absorption of minerals (calcium and phosphorus) and their use in building bones and teeth	Vitamin D-fortified milk, margarine and cereals, fish-liver oil, ultraviolet rays of sunshine on skin
E	Helps use of some vitamins and fats; protects body substances	Salad oils (cottonseed, soy, corn, peanut, sunflower), margarine, whole-grain breads and cereals, dark green leafy vegetables, nuts, dried peas and beans
K	Helps blood clot	Spinach, cabbage, cauliflower, liver

VITAMIN SUPPLEMENTS, *see* Multivitamin/mineral supplements

VOMITING refers to forced expulsion of stomach contents through the mouth. It can be caused by too much alcohol, caffeine, an infection or food poisoning. Vomiting results in weakness, mild dehydration and the lowering of some vital body elements—sodium, magnesium, chloride. There also may be severe gas which will pass in time.

Vomiting is the way the body rids itself of something irritating. Do not eat anything immediately after vomiting; just relax and give the digestive tract a chance to rest. After an hour try a little water. If this stays down slowly try other drinks, crackers, dry toast and dry cereal. For the next twenty-four hours eat simple foods like bananas, applesauce, rice and pasta. Don't drink milk; it may cause gas and diarrhea in an already irritated stomach.

W

WATER is a colorless, nearly odorless and tasteless liquid with the chemical composition H_2O. Water is essential for life. You can go for long periods without food but only for a few days without water. Your body is about two-thirds water, with water making up 83 percent of your blood, 75 percent of your muscle, 74 percent of your brain and 22 percent of your bones. Water aids in digestion, lubricates the joints, cools the body through perspiration and carries away waste in the sweat and urine.

Water has no calories but is necessary as a solvent inside and outside the cells. Thirst should ensure that water intake meets water needs. As one ages, however, thirst is not always a reliable indicator of need.

It is recommended that adults drink 6 to 8 cups of fluid a day. Most drinks are mainly water, as is much of the food we eat. Some fruits—for example, nectarines, peaches and plums—are 90 percent water. Lettuce is 95 percent water and most meats are about half water and even bread is one third water. Totaling food and drink, most adults consume and excrete about two-and-half to three quarts of water a day. This amount will increase during pregnancy, hot weather, heavy exercise and illness.

See Mineral water

WATER PILLS, *see* Diuretics

WAX is found naturally in apple skins and is responsible for their shine. Other fruits and vegetables are often *waxed*. This wax serves as a way of applying substances that help keep the produce fresh. These added waxes are similar to those used on floors but according to the Food and Drug Administration they are not harmful if eaten in small amounts. Although the waxes used on fresh produce are listed by growers and packers, this information is not displayed for consumers to see. Peeling the fruit or vegetable is the only way to remove the wax.

WEANING means to move gradually from one type of feeding to another. It usually refers to changing the infant from breast feeding to bottle or cup feeding. Patients in a hospital can be *weaned* from liquid diets to regular food and the term is applied when someone is gradually taken off a respirator until he is breathing independently once again.

WEIGHT LOSS refers to a loss of body weight. This can be accomplished through dieting, increased exercise or may be the result of illness. Every pound of weight represents 3,500 Calories that were not eaten because the person cut down on their food intake or the energy (Calories) was burned up faster than was replaced. Illness also can reduce calorie intake.

See Diets

WEIGHT WATCHERS is a self-help weight control group that meets regularly for the purpose of mutual support to accomplish weight loss. Each group has a leader, requires a dues payment, sets a weight goal for the member, and weighs members regularly. The foundation of the Weight Watchers diet is based on the

Prudent Diet set up many years ago by the New York City Department of Health. The founder of Weight Watchers, Jean Niedeitch, was successful in losing weight on this plan and she developed it into a program to help others. This diet is low in calories but balanced in needed nutrients. It is a healthy diet to follow with adjustments for quick weight loss to start and maintenance plans to keep the weight off once it has been lost.

There are other groups, similar to Weight Watchers, that offer mutual support to dieters. Some groups, however, do not have healthy dieting plans. Before joining a weight loss group check to be sure the eating plan is healthy (Calories shouldn't be under 1,000 per day) and the selection of food is varied.

See Diets, Low calorie diets, Weight loss

WHEAT GERM is the embryo of the wheat seed. It is rich in B vitamins, vitamin E and protein; one tablespoon contains 102 Calories. Wheat germ oil is extracted from wheat germ meal. It is rich in vitamin E.

WHOLE GRAIN refers to a grain, such as rice, wheat or corn, that retains its outside layers (except the chaff) and embryo portion. The germ (embryo), bran (outer layer) and endosperm are used in whatever product is being made, such as flour or cereal.

The germ is the nutrient-rich part of the grain which allows the grain to sprout and grow. The bran is the fibrous coating of the grain, rich in fiber and minerals. The endosperm is the starchy, relatively nutrient-free bulk of the grain. It is used to make refined flour.

See Refined

WHOLE WHEAT, or graham, flour is made from the entire wheat kernel including the germ, endosperm and bran. It is rich in fiber and nutrients not found in refined wheat flour made from only the endosperm. Cracked or crushed wheat is the whole grain broken into coarser fragments. Whole wheat is approximately 12 percent protein, 2 percent fat, 2 percent fiber (found mostly in the bran), 70 percent carbohydrate (found mostly in the endosperm) and 2 percent minerals (found mostly in the germ). Besides whole wheat flour, other commonly used whole wheat products are bulgur, puffed wheat, shredded wheat, cracked wheat, rolled wheat and couscous.

WINE refers to the fermented juice of the grape. If other fruit juices are used to make wine, the name of the fruit must precede the word wine. Some historians believe that primitive, cave-dwelling people may have enjoyed the fermented juices of spoiled wild berries long before grapes were ever cultivated. Archaeologists have found evidence of wine making in the middle east dating back 6,000 to 7,000 years. Egyptians were the first to realize that wines kept better in cool places and dug the first wine cellars. Wine as a beverage is found in most cultures. It may be used as a medicine, in religious ceremonies, or drunk for enjoyment. Wine consumption in the United States has been increasing recently as the consumption of distilled spirits declines.

Wine can be used as an appetite stimulant, a relaxant, and it may aid in the absorption of certain minerals. In some people who chronically take in excessive amounts of wine, iron overload can be a problem. It is generally felt that small amounts of wine are acceptable for the diabetic and may prove beneficial against heart disease. Wine's major contribution to the diet comes in the form of calories dessert wines have 175 to 200 Calories in 4 ounces; tables wines have 80 to 100 Calories in the same amount.

X

XYLITOL is a sugar alcohol of xylose, made from birchwood chips, berries, leaves or mushrooms. Xylitol is almost as sweet as table sugar (sucrose), producing a cool aftertaste when eaten. This sugar cannot be fermented by oral bacteria, therefore it does not promote tooth decay. The Food and Drug Administration has approved it for limited use in the United States in special dietary foods and chewing gum. Large doses may cause diarrhea. Some research has suggested that xylitol may be a carcinogen. Until this issue is resolved, this sugar cannot be widely used in foods.

See Carcinogen, Dental disease

Y

304 / POCKET ENCYCLOPEDIA OF NUTRITION

YEAST INFECTIONS. see Candidiasis

YELLOW: see Artificial Colors, Food Additives

YOGURT is cultured milk...

YEAST is a fungus, available commercially as brewer's yeast, baker's yeast and torula yeast.

Brewer's yeast, a by-product of brewing beer and ale, is nonfermentable, used primarily as a supplemental source of B vitamins (except for vitamin B_{12}), minerals and protein. One tablespoon provides 28 Calories and 3.9 grams of protein. Its bitter taste is the major drawback.

Baker's yeast is fermentable, available dry or compressed. It is used to leaven baked products.

Torula yeast is sold in tablets or as a powder. It is cultivated especially as a food supplement providing protein, B vitamins (including vitamin B_{12}) and minerals in a tasteless form. One tablespoon provides 28 Calories and 3.9 grams of protein.

Many who take yeast supplements find that they develop excessive, uncomfortable, embarassing gas. Start by using ½ teaspoon or less, gradually working up to a maximum daily supplement of no more than one tablespoon.

YEAST INFECTIONS, *see* Candidiasis

YELLOW #5, *see* Artificial Colors, Food allergies, MSG

YOGURT is one of the oldest fermented milks known; custardlike, it is eaten with a spoon. It is widely eaten in the middle east, and is currently popular in Europe and the United States, because people believe it makes them live longer. Yogurt has been used to smooth wrinkles, as a vaginal douche and as a cure for insomnia. Yogurt is a tasty nutritious food, with all the nutrients found in the milk from which it was made. It is not, however, a cure-all or magical food. Beware of frozen and fruit flavored yogurts; they have lots of calories!

YUCCA (cassava, manioc) is the third leading vegetable crop in the world. Yucca, more commonly called cassava, may be eaten as a starchy vegetable or ground into tapioca flour used for pudding and as a thickener. All varieties of cassava contain *linamarin,* a substance that is converted into the toxicant prussic acid by enzyme action. For this reason, the cassava root should never be eaten raw. Nutritionally, the cassava provides mainly carbohydrate with a trace of protein and a very small amount of phosphorus, calcium and iron. Yucca extract has been touted as a cure for arthritis, but scientific evidence does not support this claim.

Z

ZEN MACROBIOTICS describes both a way of eating and a way of life. *Zen* refers to meditation and *macrobiotic,* popularized by George Ohsawa, suggests long life. The Zen philosophy is ancient, from India to China and arriving in Japan in the tenth century. Zen attempts to discipline the mind so that the individual achieves a "large awareness" of the inner workings of his body.

Zen macrobiotic cooking is based on ten phases of the same diet plan. To achieve a happy, harmonious life, the person should attempt to progress from the lowest, most varied diet, -3, to the highest or purest diet, $+7$, consisting exclusively of brown rice.

Brown rice is considered a perfect food, containing a balance of yin and yang forces. All foods are classified yin (female) or yang (male). Ideal balance is five parts yin to one part yang. Brown rice contains this perfect balance and is a principal food in all the diet stages finally becoming the only food eaten in the ultimate stage. All stages encourage fluid restriction.

Overzealous followers who insist on following the rigid diet stages are in danger of malnutrition. Infants, children and pregnant women are in the most jeopardy. Brown rice is lacking vitamins A, C and B_{12} and low in calcium, iron and protein. A pound, after cooking, provides 1,190 Calories—chewy and filling but hardly nutritionally adequate. Numerous reports of scurvy, anemia, protein malnutrition, slowed growth, rickets, kidney damage and even death have been attributed to the Zen macrobiotic diet.

Using the initial stages of the diet and taking adequate fluids is similar to many other vegetarian plans but the higher, more restrictive, Zen diets could be hazardous to good health.

See Vegetarianism

Ten Stages of the Zen Macrobiotic Diet*

Stage	Cereal	Vegetables	Soup	Animal	Fruits and Salads	Desserts
			Percent of Diet			
−3	10	30	10	30	15	5
−2	20	30	10	25	10	5
−1	30	30	10	20	10	
+1	40	30	10	20	10	
+2	50	30	10	10		
+3	60	30	10			
+4	70	20	10			
+5	80	20				
+6	90	10				
+7	100					

*All stages encourage the restricted use of drinking liquids

ZINC This mineral was first isolated over a hundred years ago but wasn't known to be essential for humans until the early 1960s. The Recommended Daily Allowance for adults is 15 mg. The average American diet provides 8 to 15 mg per day but vegetarian or low protein diets may contain less. Taking zinc is becoming increasingly popular. Fifteen mg per day is not harmful but large doses of zinc can be toxic and interfere with the use of other minerals. Zinc overdoses can cause nausea, stomach pain, dizziness, anemia and kidney failure.

The human body contains about one half teaspoon (2.2 grams) of zinc with the higher amounts found in the skin, hair, nails, eyes and prostate gland; traces are found in the liver, bones and blood. Alcoholics, crash dieters and strict vegetarians are those at risk for a zinc deficiency. Since zinc is involved with the growth of the sex glands, delayed sexual development and

Food Sources of Zinc

Food	Amount	Milligrams of Zinc
Oysters, Atlantic	1 ounce	25
Beef	3 ounces	5
Lamb	3 ounces	4
Oysters, Pacific	1 ounce	3
Beans, boiled	1 cup	2
Clams, raw	4 to 5	1
Chicken, drumstick	1	1
Tuna	½ cup	1
Milk	1 cup	1
Yogurt	1 cup	1
Lentils	½ cup	1
Frankfurter	1	1
Wheat germ	1 tablespoon	1
40% Bran Flakes	1 ounce	1
Bagel	1	.5
Whole wheat bread	1 slice	.5
Oatmeal	½ cup	.5
Peanut butter	1 tablespoon	.5

stunted growth have been seen in populations who have taken in too little zinc over long periods.

Recent reports on zinc have encouraged more people to take this mineral. It may help to restore taste and smell, aid in wound healing and may be useful for those with sickle cell anemia. One recent report suggested zinc gluconate lozenges helped treat the common cold. If you are considering a zinc supplement, keep the dose below 45 mg a day.

See Minerals

APPENDIX

**Nutritive Values of the
Edible Part of Foods**

FOOD	Approximate Measures. Units. or Weight	Weight (g)	Water (%)	Food Energy (C)	Protein (g)	Fat (g)
Dairy products						
Butter. See Fats, oils; related products.						
Cheese:						
Natural:						
Blue	1 oz	28	42	100	6	8
Camembert (3 wedges per 4-oz container)	1 wedge	38	52	115	8	9
Cheddar:						
Cut pieces	1 oz	28	37	115	7	9
	1 cu. in.	17.2	37	70	4	6
Shredded	1 c	113	37	455	28	37
Cottage (curd not pressed down):						
Creamed (cottage cheese, 4% fat):						
Large curd	1 c	225	79	235	28	10
Small curd	1 c	210	79	220	26	9
Low fat (2%)	1 c	226	79	205	31	4
Low fat (1%)	1 c	226	82	165	28	2
Uncreamed (dry curd, less than 1/2% fat)	1 c	145	80	125	25	1
Cream	1 oz	28	54	100	2	10
Mozzarella, made with—						
Whole milk	1 oz	28	48	90	6	7
Part skim milk	1 oz	28	49	80	8	5
Parmesan, grated						
Cup, not pressed down	1 c	100	18	455	42	30
Tablespoon	1 T	5	18	25	2	2
Ounce	1 oz	28	18	130	12	9
Provolone	1 oz	28	41	100	7	8
Ricotta, made with—						
Whole milk	1 c	246	72	430	28	32
Part skim milk	1 c	246	74	340	28	19
Romano	1 oz	28	31	110	9	8
Swiss	1 oz	28	37	105	8	8
Pasteurized process cheese:						
American	1 oz	28	39	105	6	9
Swiss	1 oz	28	42	95	7	7
Pasteurized process cheese food, American	1 oz	28	43	95	6	7
Pasteurized process cheese spread, American	1 oz	28	48	80	5	6
Cream, sour	1 c	230	71	495	7	48
	1 T	12	71	25	Trace	3
Cream, sweet:						
Half-and-half (cream and milk)	1 c	242	81	315	7	28
	1 T	15	81	20	Trace	2

NOTE: dashes (—) denote lack of reliable data for a constituent believed to be present in measurable amount. Footnotes for this table can be found on pp. 364–66.

NUTRIENTS IN INDICATED QUANTITY

| FATTY ACIDS | | | | | | | | | | | | |
Saturated (Total) (g)	Unsaturated Oleic (g)	Unsaturated Linoleic (g)	Carbohydrate (g)	Calcium (mg)	Phosphorus (mg)	Iron (mg)	Potassium (mg)	Vitamin A Value (IU)	Vitamin B1 (mg)	Vitamin B2 (mg)	Niacin (mg)	Vitamin C (mg)
5.3	1.9	0.2	1	150	110	0.1	73	200	0.01	0.11	0.3	0
5.8	2.2	0.2	Trace	147	132	0.1	71	350	0.01	0.19	0.2	0
6.1	2.1	0.2	Trace	204	145	0.2	28	300	0.01	0.11	Trace	0
3.7	1.3	0.1	Trace	124	88	0.1	17	180	Trace	0.06	Trace	0
24.2	8.5	0.7	1	815	579	0.8	111	1,200	0.03	0.42	0.1	0
6.4	2.4	0.2	6	135	297	0.3	190	370	0.05	0.37	0.3	Trace
6.0	2.2	0.2	6	126	277	0.3	177	340	0.04	0.34	0.3	Trace
2.8	1.0	0.1	8	155	340	0.4	217	160	0.05	0.42	0.3	Trace
1.5	0.5	0.1	6	138	302	0.3	193	80	0.05	0.37	0.3	Trace
0.4	0.1	Trace	3	46	151	0.3	47	40	0.04	0.21	0.2	0
6.2	2.4	0.2	1	23	30	0.3	34	400	Trace	0.06	Trace	0
4.4	1.7	0.2	1	163	117	0.1	21	260	Trace	0.08	Trace	0
3.1	1.2	0.1	1	207	149	0.1	27	180	0.01	0.10	Trace	0
19.1	7.7	0.3	4	1,376	807	1.0	107	700	0.05	0.39	0.3	0
1.0	0.4	Trace	Trace	69	40	Trace	5	40	Trace	0.02	Trace	0
5.4	2.2	0.1	1	390	229	0.3	30	200	0.01	0.11	0.1	0
4.8	1.7	0.1	1	214	141	0.1	39	230	0.01	0.09	0.1	0
20.4	7.1	0.7	7	509	389	0.9	257	1,210	0.03	0.48	0.3	0
12.1	4.7	0.5	13	669	449	1.1	308	1,060	0.05	0.46	0.2	0
—	—	—	1	302	215	—	—	160	—	0.11	Trace	0
5.0	1.7	0.2	1	272	171	Trace	31	240	0.01	0.10	Trace	0
5.6	2.1	0.2	Trace	174	211	0.1	46	340	0.01	0.10	Trace	0
4.5	1.7	0.1	1	219	216	0.2	61	230	Trace	0.08	Trace	0
4.4	1.7	0.1	2	163	130	0.2	79	260	0.01	0.13	Trace	0
3.8	1.5	0.1	1	159	202	0.1	69	220	0.0	0.12	Trace	0
30.0	12.1	1.1	10	268	195	0.1	331	1,820	0.08	0.34	0.2	2
1.6	0.6	0.1	1	14	10	Trace	17	90	Trace	0.02	Trace	Trace
17.3	7.0	0.6	10	254	230	0.2	314	260	0.08	0.36	0.2	2
1.1	0.4	Trace	1	16	14	Trace	19	20	0.01	0.02	Trace	Trace

FOOD	Approximate Measures, Units, or Weight	Weight (g)	Water (%)	Food Energy (C)	Protein (g)	Fat (g)
Light, coffee, or table	1 c	240	74	470	6	46
	1 T	15	74	30	Trace	3
Whipped topping (pressurized)	1 c	60	61	155	2	13
	1 T	3	61	10	Trace	1
Whipping, unwhipped (volume about double when whipped):						
Heavy	1 c	238	58	820	5	88
	1 T	15	58	80	Trace	6
Light	1 c	239	64	700	5	74
	1 T	15	64	45	Trace	5
Cream products, imitation (made with vegetable fat):						
Sour dressing (imitation sour cream) made with nonfat dry milk	1 c	235	75	415	8	39
	1 T	12	75	20	Trace	2
Sweet:						
Creamers:						
Liquid (frozen)	1 c	245	77	335	2	24
	1 T	15	77	20	Trace	1
Powdered	1 c	94	2	515	5	33
	1 t	2	2	10	Trace	1
	1 T	4	50	15	Trace	1
Powdered, made with whole milk	1 c	80	67	150	3	10
	1 T	4	67	10	Trace	Trace
Pressurized	1 c	70	60	185	1	16
	1 T	4	60	10	Trace	1
Ice cream. See Milk desserts, frozen.						
Ice milk. See Milk desserts, frozen.						
Milk:						
Fluid:						
Whole (3.3% fat)	1 c	244	88	150	8	8
Lowfat (2%):						
No milk solids added	1 c	244	89	120	8	5
Milk solids added:						
Label claim less than 10 g of protein per cup	1 c	245	89	125	9	5
Label claim 10 or more grams of protein per cup (protein fortified)	1 c	246	88	135	10	5
Lowfat (1%):						
Milk solids added:						
Label claim less than 10 g of protein per cup	1 c	245	90	105	9	2
Label claim 10 or more grams of protein per cup (protein fortified)	1 c	246	89	120	10	3
No milk solids added	1 c	244	90	100	8	3

312

| FATTY ACIDS | | | | | | | | | | | | |
Saturated (Total) (g)	Unsaturated Oleic (g)	Unsaturated Linoleic (g)	Carbohydrate (g)	Calcium (mg)	Phosphorus (mg)	Iron (mg)	Potassium (mg)	Vitamin A Value (IU)	Vitamin B1 (mg)	Vitamin B2 (mg)	Niacin (mg)	Vitamin C (mg)
28.8	11.7	1.0	9	231	192	0.1	292	1,730	0.08	0.36	0.1	2
1.8	0.7	0.1	1	14	12	Trace	18	110	Trace	0.02	Trace	Trace
8.3	3.4	0.3	7	61	54	Trace	88	550	0.02	0.04	Trace	0
0.4	0.2	Trace	Trace	3	3	Trace	4	30	Trace	Trace	Trace	0
54.8	22.4	2.0	7	154	149	0.1	179	3,500	0.05	0.26	0.1	1
3.5	1.4	0.1	Trace	10	9	Trace	11	200	Trace	0.02	Trace	Trace
46.2	18.3	1.5	7	166	146	0.1	231	2,690	0.06	0.30	0.1	1
2.9	1.1	0.1	Trace	10	9	Trace	15	170	Trace	0.02	Trace	Trace
31.2	4.4	1.1	11	266	205	0.1	380	20[1]	0.09	0.38	0.2	2
1.6	0.2	0.1	1	14	10	Trace	19	Trace[1]	0.01	0.02	Trace	Trace
22.8	0.3	Trace	28	23	157	0.1	467	220[1]	0	0	0	0
1.4	Trace	0	2	1	10	Trace	29	10[1]	0	0	0	0
30.6	0.9	Trace	52	21	397	0.1	763	190[1]	0	0.16[1]	0	0
0.7	Trace	0	1	Trace	8	Trace	16	Trace[1]	0	Trace	0	0
16.3	1.0	0.2	17	5	6	0.1	14	650[1]	0	0	0	0
0.9	0.1	Trace	1	Trace	Trace	Trace	1	30[1]	0	0	0	0
8.5	0.6	0.1	13	72	69	Trace	121	290[1]	0.02	0.09	Trace	1
0.4	Trace	Trace	1	4	3	Trace	6	10[1]	Trace	Trace	Trace	Trace
13.2	1.4	0.2	11	4	13	Trace	13	330[1]	0	0	0	0
0.8	0.1	Trace	1	Trace	1	Trace	1	20[1]	0	0	0	0
5.1	2.1	0.2	11	291	228	0.1	370	310[2]	0.09	0.40	0.2	2
2.9	1.2	0.1	12	297	232	0.1	377	500	0.10	0.40	0.2	2
2.9	1.2	0.1	12	313	245	0.1	397	500	0.10	0.42	0.2	2
3.0	1.2	0.1	14	352	276	0.1	447	500	0.11	0.48	0.2	2
1.5	0.6	0.1	12	313	245	0.1	397	500	0.10	0.42	0.2	2
1.8	0.7	0.1	14	349	273	0.1	444	500	0.11	0.47	0.2	3
1.6	0.7	0.1	12	300	235	0.1	381	500	0.10	0.41	0.2	2

FOOD	Approximate Measures. Units. or Weight	Weight (g)	Water (%)	Food Energy (C)	Protein (g)	Fat (g)
Nonfat (skim):						
Milk solids added:						
Label claim less than 10 g of protein per cup	1 c	245	90	90	9	1
Label claim 10 or more grams of protein per cup (protein fortified)	1 c	246	89	100	10	1
No milk solids added	1 c	245	91	85	8	Trace
Buttermilk	1 c	245	90	100	8	2
Canned:						
Evaporated, unsweetened:						
Whole milk	1 c	252	74	340	17	19
Skim milk	1 c	255	79	200	19	1
Sweetened, condensed	1 c	306	27	980	24	27
Dried:						
Buttermilk	1 c	120	3	465	41	7
Nonfat instant:						
Envelopes	3.2 oz (net weight)	91	4	325	32	1
Cup	1 c	68[7]	4	245	24	Trace
Milk beverages:						
Chocolate milk (commercial):						
Regular	1 c	250	82	210	8	8
Lowfat (2%)	1 c	250	84	180	8	5
Lowfat (1%)	1 c	250	85	160	8	3
Eggnog (commercial)	1 c	254	74	340	10	19
Malted milk, home-prepared with 1 c of whole milk and 2 to 3 heaping teaspoons of malted milk powder (about ¾ oz)						
Chocolate	1 c of milk plus ¾ oz of powder	265	81	235	9	9
Natural	1 c of milk plus ¾ oz of powder	265	81	235	11	10
Shakes, thick:[8]						
Chocolate, container	10.6 oz	300	72	355	9	8
Vanilla, container	11 oz	313	74	350	12	9
Milk desserts, frozen:						
Ice cream:						
Regular (about 11% fat):						
Hardened	½ gal	1,064	61	2,155	38	115
	1 c	133	61	270	5	14
	3-fl-oz container	50	61	100	2	5
Soft serve (frozen custard)	1 c	173	60	375	7	23
Rich (about 16% fat), hardened	½ gal	1,188	59	2,805	33	190
	1 c	148	59	350	4	24
Ice milk:						
Hardened (about 4.3% fat)	½ gal	1,048	69	1,470	41	45
	1 c	131	69	185	5	6
Soft serve (about 2.6% fat)	1 c	175	70	225	8	5

NUTRIENTS IN INDICATED QUANTITY

Saturated (Total) (g)	Oleic (g)	Linoleic (g)	Carbohydrate (g)	Calcium (mg)	Phosphorus (mg)	Iron (mg)	Potassium (mg)	Vitamin A Value (IU)	Vitamin B1 (mg)	Vitamin B2 (mg)	Niacin (mg)	Vitamin C (mg)
	Unsaturated											
0.4	0.1	Trace	12	316	255	0.1	418	500	0.10	0.43	0.2	2
0.4	0.1	Trace	14	352	275	0.1	446	500	0.11	0.48	0.2	3
0.3	0.1	Trace	12	247	247	0.1	406	500	0.09	0.34	0.2	2
1.3	0.5	Trace	12	285	219	0.1	371	80^3	0.08	0.38	0.1	2
11.6	5.3	0.4	25	657	510	0.5	764	610^3	0.12	0.80	0.5	5
0.3	0.1	Trace	29	738	497	0.7	845	$1,000^3$	0.11	0.79	0.4	3
16.8	6.7	0.7	166	868	775	0.6	1,136	$1,000^3$	0.28	1.27	0.6	8
4.3	1.7	0.2	59	1,421	1,119	0.4	1,910	260^3	0.47	1.90	1.1	7
0.4	0.1	Trace	47	1,120	896	0.3	1,552	$2,160^6$	0.38	1.59	0.8	5
0.3	0.1	Trace	35	837	670	0.2	1,160	$1,610^6$	0.28	1.19	0.6	4
5.3	2.2	0.2	26	280	251	0.6	417	300^3	0.09	0.41	0.3	2
3.1	1.3	0.1	26	284	254	0.6	422	500	0.10	0.42	0.33	2
1.5	0.7	0.1	26	287	257	0.6	426	500	0.10	0.40	0.2	2
11.3	5.0	0.6	34	330	278	0.5	420	890	0.09	0.48	0.3	4
5.5	—	—	29	304	265	0.5	500	330	0.14	0.43	0.7	2
6.0	—	—	27	347	307	0.3	529	380	0.20	0.54	1.3	2
5.0	2.0	0.2	63	396	378	0.9	672	260	0.14	0.67	0.4	0
5.9	2.4	0.2	56	457	361	0.3	572	360	0.09	0.61	0.5	0
71.3	28.8	2.6	254	1,406	1,075	1.0	2,052	4,340	0.42	2.63	1.1	6
8.9	3.6	0.3	32	176	134	0.1	257	540	0.05	0.33	0.1	1
3.4	1.4	0.1	12	66	51	Trace	96	200	0.02	0.12	0.1	Trace
13.5	5.9	0.6	38	236	199	0.4	338	790	0.08	0.45	0.2	1
118.3	47.8	4.3	256	1,213	927	0.8	1,771	7,200	0.36	2.27	0.9	5
14.7	6.0	0.5	32	151	115	0.1	221	900	0.04	0.28	0.1	1
28.1	11.3	1.0	232	1,409	1,035	1.5	2,117	1,710	0.61	2.78	0.9	6
3.5	1.4	0.1	29	176	129	0.1	265	210	0.08	0.35	0.1	1
2.9	1.2	0.1	38	274	202	0.3	412	180	0.12	0.54	0.2	1

FOOD	Approximate Measures. Units. or Weight	Weight (g)	Water (%)	Food Energy (C)	Protein (g)	Fat (g)
Sherbet (about 2% fat)	½ gal	1,542	66	2,160	17	31
	1 c	193	66	270	2	4
Milk desserts, other:						
Custard, baked	1 c	265	77	305	14	15
Puddings:						
From home recipe:						
Starch base:						
Chocolate	1 c	260	66	385	8	12
Vanilla (blancmange)	1 c	255	76	285	9	10
Tapioca cream	1 c	165	72	220	8	8
From mix (chocolate) and milk:						
Regular (cooked)	1 c	260	70	320	9	8
Instant	1 c	260	69	325	8	7
Yogurt:						
With added milk solids:						
Made with lowfat milk:						
Fruit-flavored[9]	8 oz	227	75	230	10	3
Plain	8 oz	227	85	145	12	4
Made with nonfat milk	8 oz	227	85	125	13	Trace
Without added milk solids:						
Made with whole milk	8 oz	227	88	140	8	7
Eggs						
Eggs, large (24 oz per dozen):						
Raw:						
Whole, without shell	1	50	75	80	6	6
White	1	33	88	15	3	Trace
Yolk	1	17	49	65	3	6
Cooked, whole:						
Fried in butter	1	46	72	85	5	6
Hard-cooked, shell removed	1	50	75	80	6	6
Poached	1	50	74	80	6	6
Scrambled (milk added) in butter (also omelet	1	64	76	95	6	7
Fats, Oils; related products						
Butter:						
Regular (1 brick or 4 sticks per pound)						
Stick (½ c)	1 stick	113	16	815	1	92
Tablespoon (about ⅛ stick)	1 T	14	16	100	Trace	12
Pat (1-in. square, ⅓ in. high; 90 per pound)	1 pat	5	16	35	Trace	4
Whipped (6 sticks or two 8-oz containers per pound)						
Stick (½ c)	1 stick	76	16	540	1	61
Tablespoon (about ⅛ stick)	1 T	9	16	65	Trace	8
Pat (1¼ in. square, ⅓ in. high; 120 per pound)	1 pat	4	16	25	Trace	3

316

Saturated (Total) (g)	Unsaturated Oleic (g)	Linoleic (g)	Carbohydrate (g)	Calcium (mg)	Phosphorus (mg)	Iron (mg)	Potassium (mg)	Vitamin A Value (IU)	Vitamin B1 (mg)	Vitamin B2 (mg)	Niacin (mg)	Vitamin C (mg)
19.0	7.7	0.7	469	827	594	2.5	1,585	1,480	0.26	0.71	1.0	31
2.4	1.0	0.1	59	103	74	0.3	198	190	0.03	0.09	0.1	4
6.8	5.4	0.7	29	297	310	1.1	387	930	0.11	0.50	0.3	1
7.6	3.3	0.3	67	250	255	1.3	445	390	0.05	0.36	0.3	1
6.2	2.5	0.2	41	298	232	Trace	352	410	0.08	0.41	0.3	2
4.1	2.5	0.5	28	173	180	0.7	223	480	0.07	0.30	0.3	2
4.3	2.6	0.2	59	265	247	0.8	354	340	0.05	0.39	0.3	2
3.6	2.2	0.3	63	374	237	1.3	335	340	0.08	0.39	0.3	2
1.8	0.6	0.1	42	343	269	0.2	439	120[10]	0.08	0.40	0.2	1
2.3	0.8	0.1	16	415	326	0.2	531	150[10]	0.10	0.49	0.3	2
0.3	0.1	Trace	17	452	355	0.2	579	20[10]	0.11	0.53	0.3	2
4.8	1.7	0.1	11	274	215	0.1	351	280	0.07	0.32	0.2	1
1.7	2.0	0.6	1	28	90	1.0	65	260	0.04	0.15	Trace	0
0	0	0	Trace	4	4	Trace	45	0	Trace	0.09	Trace	0
1.7	2.1	0.6	Trace	26	86	0.9	15	310	0.04	0.07	Trace	0
2.4	2.2	0.6	1	26	80	0.9	58	290	0.03	0.13	Trace	0
1.7	2.0	0.6	1	28	90	1.0	65	260	0.04	0.14	Trace	0
1.7	2.0	0.6	1	28	90	1.0	65	260	0.04	0.13	Trace	0
2.8	2.3	0.6	1	47	97	0.9	85	310	0.04	0.16	Trace	0
57.3	23.1	2.1	Trace	27	26	0.2	29	3,470[11]	0.01	0.04	Trace	0
7.2	2.9	0.3	Trace	3	3	Trace	4	430[11]	Trace	Trace	Trace	0
2.5	1.0	0.1	Trace	1	1	Trace	1	150[11]	Trace	Trace	Trace	0
38.2	15.4	1.4	Trace	18	17	0.1	20	2,310[11]	Trace	0.03	Trace	0
4.7	1.9	0.2	Trace	2	2	Trace	2	290[11]	Trace	Trace	Trace	0
1.9	0.8	0.1	Trace	1	1	Trace	1	120[11]	0	Trace	Trace	0

FOOD	Approximate Measures, Units. or Weight	Weight (g)	Water (%)	Food Energy (C)	Protein (g)	Fat (g)
Fats, cooking (vegetable shortenings)	1 c	200	0	1,770	0	200
	1 T	13	0	110	0	13
Lard	1 c	205	0	1,850	0	205
	1 T	13	0	115	0	13
Margarine:						
Regular (1 brick or 4 sticks per pound):						
Stick (½ c)	1 stick	113	16	815	1	92
Tablespoon (about ⅛ stick)	1 T	14	16	100	Trace	12
Pat (1-in. square, ⅓ in. high; 90 per pound)	1 pat	5	16	35	Trace	4
Soft, two 8-oz. containers per pound	8 oz	227	16	1,635	1	184
	1 T	14	16	100	Trace	12
Whipped (6 sticks per pound):						
Stick (½ c)	1 stick	76	16	545	Trace	61
Tablespoon (about ⅛ stick)	1 T	9	16	70	Trace	8
Oils, salad or cooking:						
Corn	1 c	218	0	1,925	0	218
	1 T	14	0	120	0	14
Olive	1 c	216	0	1,910	0	216
	1 T	14	0	120	0	14
Peanut	1 c	216	0	1,910	0	216
	1 T	14	0	120	0	14
Safflower	1 c	218	0	1,925	0	218
	1 T	14	0	120	0	14
Soybean oil, hydrogenated (partially hardened)	1 c	218	0	1,925	0	218
	1 T	14	0	120	0	14
Soybean-cottonseed oil blend, hydrogenated	1 c	218	0	1,925	0	218
	1 T	14	0	120	0	14
Salad dressings:						
Commercial:						
Blue cheese:						
Regular	1 T	15	32	75	1	8
Low-calorie (5 C per teaspoon)	1 T	16	84	10	Trace	1
French:						
Regular	1 T	16	39	65	Trace	6
Low-calorie (5 C per teaspoon)	1 T	16	77	15	Trace	1
Italian:						
Regular	1 T	15	28	85	Trace	9
Low-calorie (2 C per teaspoon)	1 T	15	90	10	Trace	1
Mayonnaise	1 T	14	15	100	Trace	11
Mayonnaise type:						
Regular	1 T	15	41	65	Trace	6
Low calorie (8 C per teaspoon)	1 T	16	81	20	Trace	2
Tartar sauce, regular	1 T	14	34	75	Trace	8

NUTRIENTS IN INDICATED QUANTITY

| FATTY ACIDS | | | Carbohydrate (g) | Calcium (mg) | Phosphorus (mg) | Iron (mg) | Potassium (mg) | Vitamin A Value (IU) | Vitamin B1 (mg) | Vitamin B2 (mg) | Niacin (mg) | Vitamin C (mg) |
Saturated (Total) (g)	Unsaturated Oleic (g)	Unsaturated Linoleic (g)										
48.8	88.2	48.4	0	0	0	0	0	—	0	0	0	0
3.2	5.7	3.1	0	0	0	0	0	—	0	0	0	0
81.0	83.8	20.5	0	0	0	0	0	0	0	0	0	0
5.1	5.3	1.3	0	0	0	0	0	0	0	0	0	0
16.7	42.9	24.9	Trace	27	26	0.2	29	3,750[12]	0.01	0.04	Trace	0
2.1	5.3	3.1	Trace	3	3	Trace	4	470[12]	Trace	Trace	Trace	0
0.7	1.9	1.1	Trace	1	1	Trace	1	170[12]	Trace	Trace	Trace	0
32.5	71.5	65.4	Trace	53	52	0.4	59	7,500[12]	0.01	0.08	0.1	0
2.0	4.5	4.1	Trace	3	3	Trace	4	470[12]	Trace	Trace	Trace	0
11.2	28.7	16.7	Trace	18	17	0.1	20	2,500[12]	Trace	0.03	Trace	0
1.4	3.6	2.1	Trace	2	2	Trace	2	310[12]	Trace	Trace	Trace	0
27.7	53.6	125.1	0	0	0	0	0	—	0	0	0	0
1.7	3.3	7.8	0	0	0	0	0	—	0	0	0	0
30.7	154.4	17.7	0	0	0	0	0	—	0	0	0	0
1.9	9.7	1.1	0	0	0	0	0	—	0	0	0	0
37.4	98.5	67.0	0	0	0	0	0	—	0	0	0	0
2.3	6.2	4.2	0	0	0	0	0	—	0	0	0	0
20.5	25.9	159.8	0	0	0	0	0	—	0	0	0	0
1.3	1.6	10.0	0	0	0	0	0	—	0	0	0	0
31.8	93.1	75.6	0	0	0	0	0	—	0	0	0	0
2.0	5.8	4.7	0	0	0	0	0	—	0	0	0	0
38.2	63.0	99.6	0	0	0	0	0	—	0	0	0	0
2.4	3.9	6.2	0	0	0	0	0	—	0	0	0	0
1.6	1.7	3.8	1	12	11	Trace	6	30	Trace	0.02	Trace	Trace
0.5	0.3	Trace	1	10	8	Trace	5	30	Trace	0.01	Trace	Trace
1.1	1.3	3.2	3	2	2	0.1	13	—	—	—	—	—
0.1	0.1	0.4	2	2	2	0.1	13	—	—	—	—	—
1.6	1.9	4.7	1	2	1	Trace	2	Trace	Trace	Trace	Trace	—
0.1	0.1	0.4	Trace	Trace	1	Trace	2	Trace	Trace	Trace	Trace	—
2.0	2.4	5.6	Trace	3	4	0.1	5	40	Trace	0.01	Trace	—
1.1	1.4	3.2	2	2	4	Trace	1	30	Trace	Trace	Trace	—
0.4	0.4	1.0	2	3	4	Trace	1	40	Trace	Trace	Trace	—
1.5	1.8	4.1	1	3	4	0.1	11	30	Trace	Trace	Trace	Trace

FOOD	Approximate Measures, Units, or Weight	Weight (g)	Water (%)	Food Energy (C)	Protein (g)	Fat (g)
Thousand Island:						
Regular	1 T	16	32	80	Trace	8
Low calorie (10 C per teaspoon)	1 T	15	68	25	Trace	2
Homemade:						
Cooked type[13]	1 T	16	68	25	1	2
Fish, shellfish, meat, poultry; related products						
Fish and shellfish:						
Bluefish, baked with butter or margarine	3 oz	85	68	135	22	4
Clams:						
Raw, meat only	3 oz	85	82	65	11	1
Canned, solids and liquid	3 oz	85	86	45	7	1
Crabmeat (white or king), canned, not pressed down	1 c	135	77	135	24	3
Fish stick, breaded, cooked, frozen (4 × 1 1/2 in.)	1 fish stick or 1 oz	28	66	50	5	3
Haddock, breaded, fried[14]	3 oz	85	66	140	17	5
Ocean perch, breaded, fried[14]	1 fillet	85	59	195	16	11
Oysters, raw, meat only (13–19 medium selects)	1 c	240	85	160	20	4
Salmon, pink, canned, solids and liquid	3 oz	85	71	120	17	5
Sardines, Atlantic, canned in oil, drained solids	3 oz	85	62	175	20	9
Scallops, frozen, breaded, fried, reheated	6	90	60	175	16	8
Shad, baked with butter or margarine and bacon	3 oz	85	64	170	20	10
Shrimp:						
Canned meat	3 oz	85	70	100	21	1
French fried[16]	3 oz	85	57	190	17	9
Tuna, canned in oil, drained solids	3 oz	85	61	170	24	7
Tuna salad[17]	1 c	205	70	350	30	22
Meat and meat products:						
Bacon (20 slices per pound, raw), broiled or fried, crisp	2 slices	15	8	85	4	8
Beef, canned:						
Corned beef	3 oz	85	59	185	22	10
Corned beef hash	1 c	220	67	400	19	25
Beef,[18] cooked:						
Cuts braised, simmered, or pot-roasted:						
Lean and fat (piece, 2 1/2 × 2 1/2 × 3/4 in.)	3 oz	85	53	245	23	16
Lean only	2.5 oz	72	62	140	22	5
Ground beef, broiled:						
Lean with 10% fat patty	3 oz	85	60	185	23	10
Lean with 21% fat patty	2.9 oz	82	54	235	20	17

FATTY ACIDS			Carbohydrate (g)	Calcium (mg)	Phosphorus (mg)	Iron (mg)	Potassium (mg)	Vitamin A Value (IU)	Vitamin B1 (mg)	Vitamin B2 (mg)	Niacin (mg)	Vitamin C (mg)
Saturated (Total) (g)	Unsaturated Oleic (g)	Unsaturated Linoleic (g)										
1.4	1.7	4.0	2	2	3	0.1	18	50	Trace	Trace	Trace	Trace
0.4	0.4	1.0	2	2	3	0.1	17	50	Trace	Trace	Trace	Trace
0.5	0.6	0.3	2	14	15	0.1	19	80	0.01	0.03	Trace	Trace
—	—	—	0	25	244	0.6	—	40	0.09	0.08	1.6	—
—	—	—	2	59	138	5.2	154	90	0.08	0.15	1.1	8
0.2	Trace	Trace	2	47	116	3.5	119	—	0.01	0.09	0.9	—
0.6	0.4	0.1	1	61	246	1.1	149	—	0.11	0.11	2.6	—
—	—	—	2	3	47	0.1	—	0	0.01	0.02	0.5	—
1.4	2.2	1.2	5	34	210	1.0	296	—	0.03	0.06	2.7	2
2.7	4.4	2.3	6	28	192	1.1	242	—	0.10	0.10	1.6	—
1.3	0.2	0.1	8	226	343	13.2	290	740	0.34	0.43	6.0	—
0.9	0.8	0.1	0	167^{15}	243	0.7	307	60	0.03	0.16	6.8	—
3.0	2.5	0.5	0	372	424	2.5	502	190	0.02	0.17	4.6	—
—	—	—	9	—	—	—	—	—	—	—	—	—
—	—	—	0	20	266	0.5	320	30	0.11	0.22	7.3	—
0.1	0.1	Trace	1	98	224	2.6	104	50	0.01	0.03	1.5	—
2.3	3.7	2.0	9	61	162	1.7	195	—	0.03	0.07	2.3	—
1.7	1.7	0.7	0	7	199	1.6	—	70	0.04	0.10	10.1	—
4.3	6.3	6.7	7	41	291	2.7	—	590	0.08	0.23	10.3	2
2.5	3.7	0.7	Trace	2	34	0.5	35	0	0.08	0.05	0.8	—
4.9	4.5	0.2	0	17	90	3.7	—	—	0.01	0.20	2.9	—
11.9	10.9	0.5	24	29	147	4.4	440	—	0.02	0.20	4.6	—
6.8	6.5	0.4	0	10	114	2.9	184	30	0.04	0.18	3.6	—
2.1	1.8	0.2	0	10	108	2.7	176	10	0.04	0.17	3.3	—
4.0	3.9	0.3	0	10	196	3.0	261	20	0.08	0.20	5.1	—
7.0	6.7	0.4	0	9	159	2.6	221	30	0.07	0.17	4.4	—

FOOD	Approximate Measures, Units, or Weight	Weight (g)	Water (%)	Food Energy (C)	Protein (g)	Fat (g)
Roast, oven-cooked, no liquid added:						
Relatively fat, such as rib:						
Lean and fat (2 pieces, 4⅛ × 2¼ × ¼ in.)	3 oz	85	40	375	17	33
Lean only	1.8 oz	51	57	125	14	7
Relatively lean, such as heel of round:						
Lean and fat (2 pieces, 4⅛ × 2¼ × ¼ in.)	3 oz	85	62	165	25	7
Lean only	2.8 oz	78	65	125	24	3
Steak:						
Relatively fat, such as sirloin, broiled:						
Lean and fat (piece, 2½ × 2½ × ¾in.)	3 oz	85	44	330	20	27
Lean only	2.0 oz	56	59	115	18	4
Relatively lean, such as round, braised:						
Lean and fat (piece, 4⅛ × 2¼ × ½ in.)	3 oz	85	55	220	24	13
Lean only	2.4 oz	68	61	130	21	4
Beef, dried, chipped	2½-oz	71	48	145	24	4
Beef and vegetable stew	1 c	245	82	220	16	11
Beef potpie (homemade), baked[19] (piece, ⅓ of 9-in.-diam. pie)	1 piece	210	55	515	21	30
Chili con carne with beans, canned	1 c	255	72	340	19	16
Chop suey with beef and pork (homemade)	1 c	250	75	300	26	17
Heart, beef, lean, braised	3 oz	85	61	160	27	5
Lamb, cooked:						
Chop, rib (cut 3 per pound with bone), broiled:						
Lean and fat	3.1 oz	89	43	360	18	32
Lean only	2 oz	57	60	120	16	6
Leg, roasted:						
Lean and fat (2 pieces, 4⅛ × 2¼ × ¼ in.)	3 oz	85	54	235	22	16
Lean only	2.5 oz	71	62	130	20	5
Shoulder, roasted:						
Lean and fat (3 pieces, 2½ × 2½ × ¼ in.)	3 oz	85	50	285	18	23
Lean only	2.3 oz	64	61	130	17	6
Liver, beef, fried[20] (slice, 6½ × 2⅜ × ⅜ in.)	3 oz	85	56	195	22	9
Pork, cured, cooked:						
Ham, light cure, lean and fat, roasted (2 pieces, 4⅛ × 2¼ × ¼ in.)[22]	3 oz	85	54	245	18	19
Luncheon meat:						
Boiled ham, slice	1 oz	28	59	65	5	5
Canned, spiced or unspiced:						
Slice, 3 × 2 × ½ in.	1 slice	60	55	175	9	15

NUTRIENTS IN INDICATED QUANTITY

FATTY ACIDS			Carbohydrate (g)	Calcium (mg)	Phosphorus (mg)	Iron (mg)	Potassium (mg)	Vitamin A Value (IU)	Vitamin B1 (mg)	Vitamin B2 (mg)	Niacin (mg)	Vitamin C (mg)
Saturated (Total) (g)	Unsaturated Oleic (g)	Unsaturated Linoleic (g)										
14.0	13.6	0.8	0	8	158	2.2	189	70	0.05	0.13	3.1	—
3.0	2.5	0.3	0	6	131	1.8	161	10	0.04	0.11	2.6	—
2.8	2.7	0.2	0	11	208	3.2	279	10	0.06	0.19	4.5	—
1.2	1.0	0.1	0	10	199	3.0	268	Trace	0.06	0.18	4.3	—
11.3	11.1	0.6	0	9	162	2.5	220	50	0.05	0.15	4.0	—
1.8	1.6	0.2	0	7	146	2.2	202	10	0.05	0.14	3.6	—
5.5	5.2	0.4	0	10	213	3.0	272	20	0.07	0.19	4.8	—
1.7	1.5	0.2	0	9	182	2.5	238	10	0.05	0.16	4.1	—
2.1	2.0	0.1	0	14	287	3.6	142	—	0.05	0.23	2.7	0
4.9	4.5	0.2	15	29	184	2.9	613	2,400	0.15	0.17	4.7	17
7.9	12.8	6.7	39	29	149	3.8	334	1,720	0.30	0.30	5.5	6
7.5	6.8	0.3	31	82	321	4.3	594	150	0.08	0.18	3.3	—
8.5	6.2	0.7	13	60	248	4.8	425	600	0.28	0.38	5.0	33
1.5	1.1	0.6	1	5	154	5.0	197	20	0.21	1.04	6.5	1
14.8	12.1	1.2	0	8	139	1.0	200	—	0.11	0.19	4.1	—
2.5	2.1	0.2	0	6	121	1.1	174	—	0.09	0.15	3.4	—
7.3	6.0	0.6	0	9	177	1.4	241	—	0.13	0.23	4.7	—
2.1	1.8	0.2	0	9	169	1.4	227	—	0.12	0.21	4.4	—
10.8	8.8	0.9	0	9	146	1.0	206	—	0.11	0.20	4.0	—
3.6	2.3	0.2	0	8	140	1.0	193	—	0.10	0.18	3.7	—
2.5	3.5	0.9	5	9	405	7.5	323	45,390[21]	0.22	3.56	14.0	23
6.8	7.9	1.7	0	8	146	2.2	199	0	0.40	0.15	3.1	—
1.7	2.0	0.4	0	3	47	0.8	—	0	0.12	0.04	0.7	—
5.4	6.7	1.0	1	5	65	1.3	133	0	0.19	0.13	1.8	—

FOOD	Approximate Measures, Units, or Weight	Weight (g)	Water (%)	Food Energy (C)	Protein (g)	Fat (g)
Pork, fresh, cooked:[18]						
Chop, loin (cut 3 per pound with bone), broiled:						
Lean and fat	2.7 oz	78	42	305	19	25
Lean only	2 oz	56	53	150	17	9
Roast, oven-cooked, no liquid added:						
Lean and fat (piece, 2½ × 2½ × ¾ in.)	3 oz	85	46	310	21	24
Lean only	2.4 oz	68	55	175	20	10
Shoulder cut, simmered:						
Lean and fat (3 pieces, 2½ × 2½ × ¼ in.)	3 oz	85	46	320	20	26
Lean only	2.2 oz	63	60	135	18	6
Sausages (see also Luncheon meat):						
Bologna, slice	1 oz	28	56	85	3	8
Braunschweiger, slice	1 oz	28	53	90	4	8
Brown-and-serve (10 to 11 per 8-oz package), browned	1 link	17	40	70	3	6
Deviled ham, canned	1 T	13	51	45	2	4
Frankfurter (8 per 1-lb package), cooked (reheated)	1	56	57	170	7	15
Meat, potted (beef, chicken, turkey), canned	1 T	13	61	30	2	2
Pork link (16 per 1-lb package), cooked	1 link	13	35	60	2	6
Salami:						
Dry type, slice (12 per 4-oz package)	1 slice	10	30	45	2	4
Cooked type, slice (8 per 8-oz package)	1 slice	28	51	90	5	7
Vienna sausage (7 per 4-oz can)	1	16	63	40	2	3
Veal, medium fat, cooked, bone removed:						
Cutlet (4⅛ × 2¼ × ½ in.), braised or broiled	3 oz	85	60	185	23	9
Rib (2 pieces, 4⅛ × 2¼ × ¼ in.), roasted	3 oz	85	55	230	23	14
Poultry and poultry products:						
Chicken, cooked:						
Breast, fried,[23] bones removed, ½ breast (3.3 oz with bones)	2.8 oz	79	58	160	26	5
Drumstick, fried,[23] bones removed (2 oz with bones)	1.3 oz	38	55	90	12	4
Half broiler, broiled, bones removed (10.4 oz with bones)	6.2 oz	176	71	240	42	7
Chicken, canned, boneless	3 oz	85	65	170	18	10
Chicken a la king, cooked (homemade)	1 c	245	68	470	27	34
Chicken and noodles, cooked (homemade)	1 c	240	71	365	22	18
Chicken chow main:						
Canned	1 c	250	89	95	7	Trace
Homemade	1 c	250	78	255	31	10

NUTRIENTS IN INDICATED QUANTITY

Saturated (Total) (g)	Oleic (g)	Linoleic (g)	Carbohydrate (g)	Calcium (mg)	Phosphorus (mg)	Iron (mg)	Potassium (mg)	Vitamin A Value (IU)	Vitamin B1 (mg)	Vitamin B2 (mg)	Niacin (mg)	Vitamin C (mg)
8.9	10.4	2.2	0	9	209	2.7	216	0	0.75	0.22	4.5	—
3.1	3.6	0.8	0	7	181	2.2	192	0	0.63	0.18	3.8	—
8.7	10.2	2.2	0	9	218	2.7	233	0	0.78	0.22	4.8	—
3.5	4.1	0.8	0	9	211	2.6	224	0	0.73	0.21	4.4	—
9.3	10.9	2.3	0	9	118	2.6	158	0	0.46	0.21	4.1	—
2.2	2.6	0.6	0	8	111	2.3	146	0	0.42	0.19	3.7	—
3.0	3.4	0.5	Trace	2	36	0.5	65	—	0.05	0.06	0.7	—
2.6	3.4	0.8	1	3	69	1.7	—	1,850	0.05	0.41	2.3	—
2.3	2.8	0.7	Trace	—	—	—	—	—	—	—	—	—
1.5	1.8	0.4	0	1	12	0.3	—	0	0.02	0.01	0.2	—
5.6	6.5	1.2	1	3	57	0.8	—	—	0.08	0.11	1.4	—
—	—	—	0	—	—	—	—	—	Trace	0.03	0.2	—
2.1	2.4	0.5	Trace	1	21	0.3	35	0	0.10	0.04	0.5	—
1.6	1.6	0.1	Trace	1	28	0.4	—	—	0.04	0.03	0.5	—
3.1	3.0	0.2	Trace	3	57	0.7	—	—	0.07	0.07	1.2	—
1.2	1.4	0.2	Trace	1	24	0.3	—	—	0.01	0.02	0.4	—
4.0	3.4	0.4	0	9	196	2.7	258	—	0.06	0.21	4.6	—
6.1	5.1	0.6	0	10	211	2.9	259	—	0.11	0.26	6.6	—
1.4	1.8	1.1	1	9	218	1.3	—	70	0.04	0.17	11.6	—
1.1	1.3	0.9	Trace	6	89	0.9	—	50	0.03	0.15	2.7	—
2.2	2.5	1.3	0	16	355	3.0	483	160	0.09	0.34	15.5	—
3.2	3.8	2.0	0	18	210	1.3	117	200	0.03	0.11	3.7	3
12.7	14.3	3.3	12	127	358	2.5	404	1,130	0.10	0.42	5.4	12
5.9	7.1	3.5	26	26	247	2.2	149	430	0.05	0.17	4.3	Trace
—	—	—	18	45	35	1.3	418	150	0.05	0.10	1.0	13
2.4	3.4	3.1	10	58	293	2.5	473	280	0.08	0.23	4.3	10

FOOD	Approximate Measures, Units, or Weight	Weight (g)	Water (%)	Food Energy (C)	Protein (g)	Fat (g)
Chicken potpie (homemade), baked,[19] piece (1/3 of 9-in.-diam. pie)	1 piece	232	57	545	23	31
Turkey, roasted, flesh without skin:						
Dark meat, piece, 2½ × 1⅝ × ¼ in.	4 pieces	85	61	175	26	7
Light and dark meat:						
Chopped or diced	1 c	140	61	265	44	9
Pieces (1 slice white meat, 4 × 2 × ¼ in., and 2 slices dark meat, 2½ × 1⅝ × ¼ IN.)	3 pieces	85	61	160	27	5
Light meat, piece, 4 × 2 × ¼ in.	2 pieces	85	62	150	28	3
Fruits and fruit products						
Apples, raw, unpeeled, without cores:						
2¾-in. diam. (about 3 per pound with cores)	1	138	84	80	Trace	1
3¼-in. diam. (about 2 per pound with cores)	1	212	84	125	Trace	1
Apple juice, bottled or canned[24]	1 c	248	88	120	Trace	Trace
Applesauce, canned:						
Sweetened	1 c	255	76	230	1	Trace
Unsweetened	1 c	244	89	100	Trace	Trace
Apricots:						
Raw, without pits (about 12 per pound with pits)	3	107	85	55	1	Trace
Canned in heavy syrup (halves and syrup)	1 c	258	77	220	2	Trace
Dried:						
Uncooked (28 large or 37 medium halves per cup)	1 c	130	25	340	7	1
Cooked, unsweetened, fruit and liquid	1 c	250	76	215	4	1
Apricot nectar, canned	1 c	251	85	145	1	Trace
Avocados, raw, whole, without skins and seeds:						
California, mid- and late-winter (with skin and seed, 3⅛-in. diam.; 10 oz)	1	216	74	370	5	37
Florida, late summer and fall (with skin and seed, 3⅝-in. diam.; 1 lb)	1	304	78	390	4	33
Banana, without peel (about 2.6 per pound with peel)	1	119	76	100	1	Trace
Banana flakes	1 T	6	3	20	Trace	Trace
Blackberries, raw	1 c	144	85	85	2	1
Blueberries, raw	1 c	145	83	90	1	1
Cantaloupe. See Muskmelons.						
Cherries:						
Sour (tart), red, pitted, canned, water pack	1 c	244	88	105	2	Trace
Sweet, raw, without pits and stems	10	68	80	45	1	Trace
Cranberry juice cocktail, bottled, sweetened	1 c	253	83	164	Trace	Trace
Cranberry sauce, sweetened, canned, strained	1 c	277	62	405	Trace	1

NUTRIENTS IN INDICATED QUANTITY

Saturated (Total) (g)	Oleic (g)	Linoleic (g)	Carbohydrate (g)	Calcium (mg)	Phosphorus (mg)	Iron (mg)	Potassium (mg)	Vitamin A Value (IU)	Vitamin B1 (mg)	Vitamin B2 (mg)	Niacin (mg)	Vitamin C (mg)
11.3	10.9	5.6	42	70	232	3.0	343	3,090	0.34	0.31	5.5	5
2.1	1.5	1.5	0	—	—	2.0	338	—	0.03	0.20	3.6	—
2.5	1.7	1.8	0	11	351	2.5	514	—	0.07	0.25	10.8	—
1.5	1.0	1.1	0	7	213	1.5	312	—	0.04	0.15	6.5	—
0.9	0.6	0.7	0	—	—	1.0	349	—	0.04	0.12	9.4	—
—	—	—	20	10	14	0.4	152	120	0.04	0.03	0.1	6
—	—	—	31	15	21	0.6	233	190	0.06	0.04	0.2	8
—	—	—	30	15	22	1.5	250	—	0.02	0.05	0.2	2[25]
—	—	—	61	10	13	1.3	166	100	0.05	0.03	0.1	3[25]
—	—	—	26	10	12	1.2	190	100	0.05	0.02	0.1	2[25]
—	—	—	14	18	25	0.5	301	2,890	0.03	0.04	0.6	11
—	—	—	57	28	39	0.8	604	4,490	0.05	0.05	1.0	10
—	—	—	86	87	140	7.2	1,273	14,170	0.01	0.21	4.3	16
—	—	—	54	55	88	4.5	795	7,500	0.01	0.13	2.5	8
—	—	—	37	23	30	0.5	379	2,380	0.03	0.03	0.5	36[26]
5.5	22.0	3.7	13	22	91	1.3	1,303	630	0.24	0.43	3.5	30
6.7	15.7	5.3	27	30	128	1.8	1,836	880	0.33	0.61	4.9	43
—	—	—	26	10	31	0.8	440	230	0.06	0.07	0.8	12
—	—	—	5	2	6	0.2	92	50	0.01	0.01	0.2	Trace
—	—	—	19	46	27	1.3	245	290	0.04	0.06	0.6	30
—	—	—	22	22	19	1.5	117	150	0.04	0.09	0.7	20
—	—	—	26	37	32	0.7	317	1,660	0.07	0.05	0.5	12
—	—	—	12	15	13	0.3	129	70	0.03	0.04	0.3	7
—	—	—	42	13	8	0.8	25	Trace	0.03	0.03	0.1	81[27]
—	—	—	104	17	11	0.6	83	60	0.03	0.03	0.1	6

FOOD	Approximate Measures, Units, or Weight	Weight (g)	Water (%)	Food Energy (C)	Protein (g)	Fat (g)
Dates:						
Whole, without pits	10	80	23	220	2	Trace
Chopped	1 c	178	23	490	4	1
Fruit cocktail, canned, in heavy syrup	1 c	255	80	195	1	Trace
Grapefruit:						
Raw, medium, 3¾-in. diam. (about 1 lb 1 oz):						
Pink or red, with peel	½	241[28]	89	50	1	Trace
White, with peel	½	241[28]	89	45	1	Trace
Canned, sections with syrup	1 c	254	81	180	2	Trace
Grapefruit juice:						
Raw, pink, red, or white	1 c	246	90	95	1	Trace
Canned, white:						
Unsweetened	1 c	247	89	100	1	Trace
Sweetened	1 c	250	86	135	1	Trace
Frozen, concentrate, unsweetened:						
Undiluted	6 fl oz	207	62	300	4	1
Diluted with 3 parts water by volume	1 c	246	89	100	1	Trace
Dehydrated crystals, prepared with water (1 lb yields about 1 gal)	1 c	247	90	100	1	Trace
Grapes, European type (adherent skin), raw:						
Thompson seedless	10	50	81	35	Trace	Trace
Tokay and Emperor (seeded)	10	60[30]	81	40	Trace	Trace
Grape juice:						
Canned or bottled	1 c	253	83	165	1	Trace
Frozen concentrate, sweetened:						
Undiluted	6 fl oz	216	53	395	1	Trace
Diluted with 3 parts water by volume	1 c	250	86	135	1	Trace
Grape drink, canned	1 c	250	86	135	Trace	Trace
Lemon, raw, size 165, without peel and seeds (about 4 per pound with peels and seeds)	1	74	90	20	1	Trace
Lemonade concentrate, frozen:						
Undiluted	6 fl oz	219	49	425	Trace	Trace
Diluted with 4⅓ parts water by volume	1 c	248	89	105	Trace	Trace
Lemon juice:						
Raw	1 c	244	91	60	1	Trace
Canned or bottled, unsweetened	1 c	244	92	55	1	Trace
Frozen, single strength, unsweetened	6 oz	183	92	40	1	Trace
Limeade concentrate, frozen:						
Undiluted	6 fl oz	218	50	410	Trace	Trace
Diluted with 4⅓ parts water by volume	1 c	247	89	100	Trace	Trace
Lime juice:						
Raw	1 c	246	90	65	1	Trace
Canned, unsweetened	1 c	246	90	65	1	Trace

Saturated (Total) (g)	Unsaturated Oleic (g)	Unsaturated Linoleic (g)	Carbohydrate (g)	Calcium (mg)	Phosphorus (mg)	Iron (mg)	Potassium (mg)	Vitamin A Value (IU)	Vitamin B1 (mg)	Vitamin B2 (mg)	Niacin (mg)	Vitamin C (mg)
—	—	—	58	47	50	2.4	518	40	0.07	0.08	1.8	0
—	—	—	130	105	112	5.3	1,153	90	0.16	0.18	3.9	0
—	—	—	50	23	31	1.0	411	360	0.05	0.03	1.0	5
—	—	—	13	20	20	0.5	166	540	0.05	0.02	0.2	44
—	—	—	12	19	19	0.5	159	10	0.05	0.02	0.2	44
—	—	—	45	33	36	0.8	343	30	0.08	0.05	0.5	76
—			23	22	37	0.5	399	29	0.10	0.05	0.5	93
—	—	—	24	20	35	1.0	400	20	0.07	0.05	0.5	84
—	—	—	32	20	35	1.0	405	30	0.08	0.05	0	78
—	—	—	72	70	124	0.8	1,250	60	0.29	0.12	1.4	286
—	—	—	24	25	42	0.2	420	20	0.10	0.04	0.5	96
—	—	—	24	22	40	0.2	412	20	0.10	0.05	0.5	91
—	—	—	9	6	10	0.2	87	50	0.03	0.02	0.2	2
—	—	—	10	7	11	0.2	99	60	0.03	0.02	0.2	2
—	—	—	42	28	30	0.8	293	—	0.10	0.05	0.5	Trace[25]
—	—	—	100	22	32	0.9	255	40	0.13	0.22	1.5	32[31]
—	—	—	33	8	10	0.3	85	10	0.05	0.08	0.5	10[31]
—	—	—	35	8	10	0.3	88	—	0.03[32]	0.03[32]	0.3	32
—	—	—	6	19	12	0.4	102	10	0.03	0.01	0.1	39
—	—	—	112	9	13	0.4	153	40	0.05	0.06	0.7	66
—	—	—	28	2	3	0.1	40	10	0.01	0.02	0.2	17
—	—	—	20	17	24	0.5	344	50	0.07	0.02	0.2	112
—	—	—	19	17	24	0.5	344	50	0.07	0.02	0.2	102
—	—	—	13	13	16	0.5	258	40	0.05	0.02	0.2	81
—	—	—	108	11	13	0.2	129	Trace	0.02	0.02	0.2	26
—	—	—	27	3	3	Trace	32	Trace	Trace	Trace	Trace	6
—	—	—	22	22	27	0.5	256	20	0.05	0.02	0.2	79
—	—	—	22	22	27	0.5	256	20	0.05	0.02	0.2	52

FOOD	Approximate Measures, Units, or Weight	Weight (g)	Water (%)	Food Energy (C)	Protein (g)	Fat (g)
Muskmelons, raw, with rind, without seed cavity:						
Cantaloupe, orange-fleshed (with rind and seed cavity, 5-in. diam., 2⅓ lb), with rind	½	477³³	91	80	2	Trace
Honeydew (with rind and seed cavity, 6½-in. diam., 5¼ lb), with rind	⅒	226³³	91	50	1	Trace
Oranges, all commercial varieties, raw:						
Whole, 2⅝-in. diam., without peel and seeds (about 2½ per pound with peel and seeds)	1	131	86	65	1	Trace
Sections without membranes	1 c	180	86	90	2	Trace
Orange juice:						
Raw, all varieties	1 c	248	88	110	2	Trace
Canned, unsweetened	1 c	249	87	120	2	Trace
Frozen concentrate:						
Undiluted	6 fl oz	213	55	360	5	Trace
Diluted with 3 parts water by volume	1 c	249	87	120	2	Trace
Dehydrated crystals, prepared with water (1 lb yields about 1 gal)	1 c	248	88	115	1	Trace
Orange and grapefruit juice:						
Frozen concentrate:						
Undiluted	6 fl oz	210	59	330	4	1
Diluted with 3 parts water by volume	1 c	248	88	110	1	Trace
Papayas, raw, ½-in. cubes	1 c	140	89	55	1	Trace
Peaches:						
Raw:						
Whole, 2½-in. diam., peeled, pitted (about 4 per pound with peels and pits)	1	100	89	40	1	Trace
Sliced	1 c	170	89	65	1	Trace
Canned, yellow-fleshed, solids and liquids (halves or slices):						
Syrup pack	1 c	256	79	200	1	Trace
Water pack	1 c	244	91	75	1	Trace
Dried:						
Uncooked	1 c	160	25	420	5	1
Cooked, unsweetened, halves and juice	1 c	250	77	205	3	1
Frozen, sliced, sweetened:						
10-oz container	1 container	284	77	250	1	Trace
Cup	1 c	250	77	220	1	Trace
Pears:						
Raw, with skin, cored:						
Anjou, 3-in. diam. (about 2 per pound with cores and stems)	1	200	83	120	1	1
Bartlett, 2½-in. diam. (about 2½ per pound with cores and stems)	1	164	83	100	1	1

NUTRIENTS IN INDICATED QUANTITY

Saturated (Total) (g)	Oleic (g)	Linoleic (g)	Carbohydrate (g)	Calcium (mg)	Phosphorus (mg)	Iron (mg)	Potassium (mg)	Vitamin A Value (IU)	Vitamin B1 (mg)	Vitamin B2 (mg)	Niacin (mg)	Vitamin C (mg)
—	—	—	20	38	44	1.1	682	9,240	0.11	0.08	1.6	90
—	—	—	11	21	24	0.6	374	60	0.06	0.04	0.9	34
—	—	—	16	54	26	0.5	263	260	0.13	0.05	0.5	66
—	—	—	22	74	36	0.7	360	360	0.18	0.07	0.7	90
—	—	—	26	27	42	0.5	496	500	0.22	0.07	1.0	124
—	—	—	28	25	45	1.0	496	500	0.17	0.05	0.7	100
—	—	—	87	75	126	0.9	1,500	1,620	0.68	0.11	2.8	360
—	—	—	29	25	42	0.2	503	540	0.23	0.03	0.9	120
—	—	—	27	25	40	0.5	518	500	0.20	0.07	1.0	109
—	—	—	78	61	99	0.8	1,308	800	0.48	0.06	2.3	302
—	—	—	26	20	32	0.2	439	270	0.15	0.02	0.7	102
—	—	—	14	28	22	0.4	328	2,450	0.06	0.06	0.4	78
—	—	—	10	9	19	0.5	202	1,330[34]	0.02	0.05	1.0	7
—	—	—	16	15	32	0.9	343	2,260[34]	0.03	0.09	1.7	12
—	—	—	51	10	31	0.8	33	1,100	0.03	0.05	1.5	8
—	—	—	20	10	32	0.7	334	1,100	0.02	0.07	1.5	7
—	—	—	109	77	187	9.6	1,520	6,240	0.02	0.30	8.5	29
—	—	—	54	38	93	4.8	743	3,050	0.01	0.15	3.8	5
—	—	—	64	11	37	1.4	352	1,850	0.03	0.11	2.0	116[35]
—	—	—	57	10	33	1.3	310	1,630	0.03	0.10	1.8	103[35]
—	—	—	31	16	22	0.6	260	40	0.04	0.08	0.2	8
—	—	—	25	13	18	0.5	213	30	0.03	0.07	0.2	7

FOOD	Approximate Measures, Units, or Weight	Weight (g)	Water (%)	Food Energy (C)	Protein (g)	Fat (g)
Bosc, 2½-in. diam. (about 3 per pound with cores and stems)	1	141	83	85	1	1
Canned, solids and liquids, syrup pack, heavy (halves or slices)	1 c	255	80	195	1	1
Pineapple						
Raw, diced	1 c	155	85	80	1	Trace
Canned, heavy syrup pack, solids and liquid:						
Crushed, chunks, tidbits	1 c	255	80	190	1	Trace
Slices and liquid:	1 slice; 2¼ T					
Large	liquid	105	80	80	Trace	Trace
	1 slice; 1¼ T					
Medium	liquid	58	80	45	Trace	Trace
Pineapple juice, unsweetened, canned	1 c	250	86	140	1	Trace
Plums:						
Raw, without pits:						
Japanese and hybrid (2⅛-in. diam., about 6½ per pound with pits)	1	66	87	30	Trace	Trace
Prune-type (1½-in. diam., about 15 per pound with pits)	1	28	79	20	Trace	Trace
Canned, heavy syrup pack (italian prunes), with pits and liquid:						
Cup	1 c[36]	272	77	215	1	Trace
Portion	3; 2¾ T liquid[36]	140	77	110	1	Trace
Prunes, dried, "softenized," with pits:						
Uncooked	4 extra large or 5 large	49[36]	28	110	1	Trace
Cooked, unsweetened, all sizes, fruit and liquid	1 c	250[36]	66	255	2	1
Prune juice, canned or bottled	1 c	256	80	195	1	Trace
Raisins, seedless:						
Cup, not pressed down	1 c	145	18	420	4	Trace
Packet, ½ oz (1½ T)	1 packet	14	18	40	Trace	Trace
Raspberries, red:						
Raw, capped, whole	1 c	123	84	70	1	1
Frozen, sweetened	10 oz	284	74	280	2	1
Rhubarb, cooked, added sugar:						
From raw	1 c	270	63	380	1	Trace
From frozen, sweetened	1 c	270	63	385	1	1
Strawberries:						
Raw, whole berries, capped	1 c	149	90	55	1	1
Frozen, sweetened:						
Sliced	10 oz	284	71	310	1	1
Whole	1 lb (about 1¾ c)	454	76	415	2	1
Tangerine, raw, 2⅜-in. diam., size 176, without peel (about 4 per pound with peels and seeds)	1	86	87	40	1	Trace

NUTRIENTS IN INDICATED QUANTITY

Saturated (Total) (g)	Oleic (g)	Linoleic (g)	Carbohydrate (g)	Calcium (mg)	Phosphorus (mg)	Iron (mg)	Potassium (mg)	Vitamin A Value (IU)	Vitamin B1 (mg)	Vitamin B2 (mg)	Niacin (mg)	Vitamin C (mg)
—	—	—	22	11	16	0.4	83	30	0.03	0.06	0.1	6
—	—	—	50	13	18	0.5	214	10	0.03	0.05	0.3	3
—	—	—	21	26	12	0.8	226	110	0.14	0.05	0.3	26
—	—	—	49	28	13	0.8	245	130	0.20	0.05	0.5	18
—	—	—	20	12	5	0.3	101	50	0.08	0.02	0.2	7
—	—	—	11	6	3	0.2	56	30	0.05	0.01	0.1	4
—	—	—	34	38	23	0.8	373	130	0.13	0.05	0.5	80[27]
—	—	—	8	8	12	0.3	112	160	0.02	0.02	0.3	4
—	—	—	6	3	5	0.1	48	80	0.01	0.01	0.1	1
—	—	—	56	23	26	2.3	367	3,130	0.05	0.05	1.0	5
—	—	—	29	12	13	1.2	189	1,610	0.03	0.03	0.5	3
—	—	—	29	22	34	1.7	298	690	0.04	0.07	0.7	1
—	—	—	67	51	79	3.8	695	1,590	0.07	0.15	1.5	2
—	—	—	49	36	51	1.8	602	—	0.03	0.03	1.0	5
—	—	—	112	90	146	5.1	1,106	30	0.16	0.12	0.7	1
—	—	—	11	9	14	0.5	107	Trace	0.02	0.01	0.1	Trace
—	—	—	17	27	27	1.1	207	160	0.04	0.11	1.1	31
—	—	—	70	37	48	1.7	284	200	0.06	0.17	1.7	60
—	—	—	97	211	41	1.6	548	220	0.05	0.14	0.8	16
—	—	—	98	211	32	1.9	475	190	0.03	0.11	0.5	16
—	—	—	13	31	31	1.5	244	90	0.04	0.10	0.9	88
—	—	—	79	40	48	2.0	318	90	0.06	0.17	1.4	151
—	—	—	107	59	73	2.7	472	140	0.09	0.27	2.3	249
—	—	—	10	34	15	0.3	108	360	0.05	0.02	0.1	27

FOOD	Approximate Measures. Units. or Weight	Weight (g)	Water (%)	Food Energy (C)	Protein (g)	Fat (g)
Tangerine juice, canned, sweetened	1 c	249	87	125	1	Trace
Watermelon, raw, 4 × 8 in. wedge with rind and seeds (1/16 of 32⅔-lb melon, 10 × 16 in.)	1	926[37]	93	110	2	1
Grain products						
Bagel, 3-in. diam.:						
Egg	1	55	32	165	6	2
Water	1	55	29	165	6	1
Barley, pearled, light, uncooked	1 c	200	11	700	16	2
Biscuits, baking powder, 2-in. diam. (enriched flour, vegetable shortening):						
Homemade	1	28	27	105	2	5
From mix	1	28	29	90	2	3
Bread crumbs (enriched):[38]						
Dry, grated	1 c	100	7	390	13	5
Soft. See Bread, White.						
Bread:						
Boston brown bread, canned, slice, 3¼ × ½ in.[38]	1 sl	45	45	95	2	1
Cracked wheat (¾ enriched wheat flour, ¼ cracked wheat):[38]						
Loaf	1 lb	454	35	1,195	39	10
Slice (18 per loaf)	1 sl	25	35	65	2	1
French or Vienna, enriched:[38]						
Loaf	1 lb	454	31	1,315	41	14
Slice:						
French (5 × 2½ × 1 in.)	1 sl	35	31	100	3	1
Vienna (4¾ × 4 × ½ in.)	1 sl	25	31	75	2	1
Italian, enriched:						
Loaf	1 lb	454	32	1,250	41	4
Slice, 4½ × 3¼ × ¾ in.	1 sl	30	32	85	3	Trace
Raisin, enriched:[38]						
Loaf	1 lb	454	35	1,190	30	13
Slice (18 per loaf)	1 sl	25	35	65	2	1
Rye:						
American, light (⅔ enriched wheat flour, ⅓ rye flour):						
Loaf	1 lb	454	36	1,100	41	5
Slice (4¾ × 3¾ × 7/16 in.)	1 sl	25	36	60	2	Trace
Pumpernickel (⅔ rye flour, ⅓ enriched wheat flour):						
Loaf	1 lb	454	34	1,115	41	5
Slice (5 × 4 × ⅜ in.)	1 sl	32	34	80	3	Trace

NUTRIENTS IN INDICATED QUANTITY												
FATTY ACIDS												
Saturated (Total) (g)	Unsaturated Oleic (g)	Linoleic (g)	Carbohydrate (g)	Calcium (mg)	Phosphorus (mg)	Iron (mg)	Potassium (mg)	Vitamin A Value (IU)	Vitamin B1 (mg)	Vitamin B2 (mg)	Niacin (mg)	Vitamin C (mg)
—	—	—	30	44	35	0.5	440	1,040	0.15	0.05	0.2	54
—	—	—	27	30	43	2.1	426	2,510	0.13	0.13	0.9	30
0.5	0.9	0.8	28	9	43	1.2	41	30	0.14	0.10	1.2	0
0.2	0.4	0.6	30	8	41	1.2	42	0	0.15	0.11	1.4	0
0.3	0.2	0.8	158	32	378	4.0	320	0	0.24	0.10	6.2	0
1.2	2.0	1.2	13	34	49	0.4	33	Trace	0.08	0.08	0.7	Trace
0.6	1.1	0.7	15	19	65	0.6	32	Trace	0.09	0.08	0.8	Trace
1.0	1.6	1.4	73	122	141	3.6	152	Trace	0.35	0.35	4.8	Trace
0.1	0.2	0.2	21	41	72	0.9	131	0[39]	0.06	0.04	0.7	0
2.2	3.0	3.9	236	399	581	9.5	608	Trace	1.52	1.13	14.4	Trace
0.1	0.2	0.2	13	22	32	0.5	34	Trace	0.08	0.06	0.8	Trace
3.2	4.7	4.6	251	195	386	10.0	408	Trace	1.80	1.10	15.0	Trace
0.2	0.4	0.4	19	15	30	0.8	32	Trace	0.14	0.08	1.2	Trace
0.2	0.3	0.3	14	11	21	0.6	23	Trace	0.10	0.06	0.8	Trace
0.6	0.3	1.5	256	77	349	10.0	336	0	1.80	1.10	15.0	0
Trace	Trace	0.1	17	5	23	0.7	22	0	0.12	0.07	1.0	0
3.0	4.7	3.9	243	322	395	10.0	1,057	Trace	1.70	1.07	10.7	Trace
0.2	0.3	0.2	13	18	22	0.6	58	Trace	0.09	0.06	0.6	Trace
0.7	0.5	2.2	236	340	667	9.1	658	0	1.35	0.98	12.9	0
Trace	Trace	0.1	13	19	37	0.5	36	0	0.07	0.05	0.7	0
0.7	0.5	2.4	241	381	1,039	11.8	2,059	0	1.30	0.93	8.5	0
0.1	Trace	0.2	17	27	73	0.8	145	0	0.09	0.07	0.6	0

FOOD	Approximate Measures, Units, or Weight	Weight (g)	Water (%)	Food Energy (C)	Protein (g)	Fat (g)
White, enriched:[38]						
Soft-crumb type:						
Loaf	1 lb	454	36	1,225	39	15
Slice (18 per loaf)	1 sl	25	36	70	2	1
Toast	1 sl	22	25	70	2	1
Slice (22 per loaf)	1 sl	20	36	55	2	1
Toast	1 sl	17	25	55	2	1
Loaf	1½ lb	680	36	1,835	59	22
Slice (24 per loaf)	1 sl	28	36	75	2	1
Toast	1 sl	24	25	75	2	1
Slice (28 per loaf)	1 sl	24	36	65	2	1
Toast	1 sl	21	25	65	2	1
Crumbs	1 c	45	36	120	4	1
Cubes	1 c	30	36	80	3	1
Firm-crumb type:						
Loaf	1 lb	454	35	1,245	41	17
Slice (20 per loaf)	1 sl	23	35	65	2	1
Toast	1 sl	20	24	65	2	1
Loaf	2 lb	907	35	2,495	82	34
Slice (34 per loaf)	1 sl	27	35	75	2	1
Toast	1 sl	23	24	75	2	1
Whole wheat:						
Soft-crumb type:[38]						
Loaf	1 lb	454	36	1,095	41	12
Slice (16 per loaf)	1 sl	28	36	65	3	1
Toast	1 sl	24	24	65	3	1
Firm-crumb type:[38]						
Loaf	1 lb	454	36	1,100	48	14
Slice (18 per loaf)	1 sl	25	36	60	3	1
Toast	1 sl	21	24	60	3	1
Breakfast cereals:						
Hot type, cooked:						
Corn (hominy) grits, degermed:						
Enriched	1 c	245	87	125	3	Trace
Unenriched	1 c	245	87	125	3	Trace
Farina, quick-cooking, enriched	1 c	245	89	105	3	Trace
Oatmeal or rolled oats	1 c	240	87	130	5	2
Wheat, rolled	1 c	240	80	180	5	1
Wheat, whole meal	1 c	245	88	110	4	1
Ready-to-eat:						
Bran flakes (40% bran), added sugar, salt, iron, vitamins	1 c	35	3	105	4	1
Bran flakes with raisins, added sugar, salt, iron, vitamins	1 c	50	7	145	4	1

336

FATTY ACIDS			Carbohydrate (g)	Calcium (mg)	Phosphorus (mg)	Iron (mg)	Potassium (mg)	Vitamin A Value (IU)	Vitamin B1 (mg)	Vitamin B2 (mg)	Niacin (mg)	Vitamin C (mg)
Saturated (Total) (g)	Unsaturated Oleic (g)	Linoleic (g)										
3.4	5.3	4.6	229	381	440	11.3	476	Trace	1.80	1.10	15.0	Trace
0.2	0.3	0.3	13	21	24	0.6	26	Trace	0.10	0.06	0.8	Trace
0.2	0.3	0.3	13	21	24	0.6	26	Trace	0.08	0.06	0.8	Trace
0.2	0.2	0.2	10	17	19	0.5	21	Trace	0.08	0.05	0.7	Trace
0.2	0.2	0.2	10	17	19	0.5	21	Trace	0.06	0.05	0.7	Trace
5.2	7.9	6.9	343	571	660	17.0	714	Trace	2.70	1.65	22.5	Trace
0.2	0.3	0.3	14	24	27	0.7	29	Trace	0.11	0.07	0.9	Trace
0.2	0.3	0.3	14	24	27	0.7	29	Trace	0.09	0.07	0.9	Trace
0.2	0.3	0.2	12	20	23	0.6	25	Trace	0.10	0.06	0.8	Trace
0.2	0.3	0.2	12	20	23	0.6	25	Trace	0.08	0.06	0.8	Trace
0.3	0.5	0.5	23	38	44	1.1	47	Trace	0.18	0.11	1.5	Trace
0.2	0.3	0.3	15	25	29	0.8	32	Trace	0.12	0.07	1.0	Trace
3.9	5.9	5.2	228	435	463	11.3	549	Trace	1.80	1.10	15.0	Trace
0.2	0.3	0.3	12	22	23	0.6	28	Trace	0.09	0.06	0.8	Trace
0.2	0.3	0.3	12	22	23	0.6	28	Trace	0.07	0.06	0.8	Trace
7.7	11.8	10.4	455	871	925	22.7	1,097	Trace	3.60	2.20	30.0	Trace
0.2	0.3	0.3	14	26	28	0.7	33	Trace	0.11	0.06	0.9	Trace
0.2	0.3	0.3	14	26	28	0.7	33	Trace	0.09	0.06	0.9	Trace
2.2	2.9	4.2	224	381	1,152	13.6	1,161	Trace	1.37	0.45	12.7	Trace
0.1	0.2	0.2	14	24	71	0.8	72	Trace	0.09	0.03	0.8	Trace
0.1	0.2	0.2	14	24	71	0.8	72	Trace	0.07	0.03	0.8	Trace
2.5	3.3	4.9	216	449	1,034	13.6	1,238	Trace	1.17	0.54	12.7	Trace
0.1	0.2	0.3	12	25	57	0.8	68	Trace	0.06	0.03	0.7	Trace
0.1	0.2	0.3	12	25	57	0.8	68	Trace	0.05	0.03	0.7	Trace
Trace	Trace	0.1	27	2	25	0.7	27	Trace[40]	0.10	0.07	1.0	0
Trace	Trace	0.1	27	2	25	0.2	27	Trace[40]	0.05	0.02	0.5	0
Trace	Trace	0.1	22	147	113[41]	[42]	25	0	0.12	0.07	1.0	0
0.4	0.8	0.9	23	22	137	1.4	146	0	0.19	0.05	0.2	0
—	—	—	41	19	182	1.7	202	0	0.17	0.07	2.2	0
—	—	—	23	17	127	1.2	118	0	0.15	0.05	1.5	0
—	—	—	28	19	125	5.6	137	1,540	0.46	0.52	6.2	0
—	—	—	40	28	146	7.9	154	2,200[43]	[44]	[44]	[44]	0

FOOD	Approximate Measures. Units. or Weight	Weight (g)	Water (%)	Food Energy (C)	Protein (g)	Fat (g)
Corn flakes:						
Plain, added sugar, salt, iron, vitamins	1 c	25	4	95	2	Trace
Sugar-coated, added salt, iron, vitamins	1 c	40	2	155	2	Trace
Corn, oat flour, puffed, added sugar, salt, iron, vitamins	1 c	20	4	80	2	1
Corn, shredded, added sugar, salt, iron, thiamin, niacin	1 c	25	3	95	2	Trace
Oats, puffed, added sugar, salt, minerals, vitamins	1 c	25	3	100	3	1
Rice, puffed:						
Plain, added iron, thiamin, niacin	1 c	15	4	60	1	Trace
Presweetened, added salt, iron, vitamins	1 c	28	3	115	1	0
Wheat flakes, added sugar, salt, iron, vitamins	1 c	30	4	105	3	Trace
Wheat, puffed:						
Plain, added iron, thiamin, niacin	1 c	15	3	55	2	Trace
Presweetened, added salt, iron, vitamins	1 c	38	3	140	3	Trace
Wheat, shredded, plain	1 oblong biscuit or ½ spoon-size biscuits	25	7	90	2	1
Wheat germ, without salt and sugar, toasted	1 T	6	4	25	2	1
Buckwheat flour, light, sifted	1 c	98	12	340	6	1
Bulgur, canned, seasoned	1 c	135	56	245	8	4
Cake icings. See Sugars and Sweets.						
Cakes made from cake mixes with enriched flour:[46]						
Angel food:						
Whole cake (9¾-in. diam. tube cake)	1	635	34	1,645	36	1
Piece, 1/12 of cake	1	53	34	135	3	Trace
Coffee cake:						
Whole cake (7¾ × 5⅝ × 1¼ in.)	1	430	30	1,385	27	41
Piece, 1/6 of cake	1	72	30	230	5	7
Cupcake, made with egg, milk, 2½-in. diam.:						
Without icing	1	25	26	90	1	3
With chocolate icing	1	36	22	130	2	5
Devil's food with chocolate icing:						
Whole, 2-layer cake (8- or 9-in. diam.)	1	1,107	24	3,755	49	136
Piece, 1/16 of cake	1	69	24	235	3	8
Cupcake, 2½-in. diam.	1	35	24	120	2	4
Gingerbread:						
Whole cake (8-in. square)	1	570	37	1,575	18	39
Piece, 1/9 of cake	1	63	37	175	2	4

Saturated (Total) (g)	Unsaturated Oleic (g)	Unsaturated Linoleic (g)	Carbohydrate (g)	Calcium (mg)	Phosphorus (mg)	Iron (mg)	Potassium (mg)	Vitamin A Value (IU)	Vitamin B1 (mg)	Vitamin B2 (mg)	Niacin (mg)	Vitamin C (mg)
—	—	—	21	[44]	9	[44]	30	[44]	[44]	[44]	[44]	13[45]
—	—	—	37	1	10	[44]	27	1,760	0.53	0.60	7.1	21[45]
—	—	—	16	4	18	5.7	—	880	0.26	0.30	3.5	11
—	—	—	22	1	10	0.6	—	0	0.33	0.05	4.4	13
—	—	—	19	[44]	102	4.0	—	1,100	0.33	0.38	4.4	13
—	—	—	13	3	14	0.3	15	0	0.07	0.01	0.7	0
—	—	—	26	3	14	[44]	43	1,240[45]	[44]	[44]	[44]	15[45]
—	—	—	24	12	83	4.8	81	1,320	0.40	0.45	5.3	16
—	—	—	12	4	48	0.6	51	0	0.08	0.03	1.2	0
—	—	—	33	7	52	[44]	63	1,680	0.50	0.57	6.7	20[45]
—	—	—	20	11	97	0.9	87	0	0.06	0.03	1.1	0
—	—	—	3	3	70	0.5	57	10	0.11	0.05	0.3	1
0.2	0.4	0.4	78	11	86	1.0	314	0	0.08	0.04	0.4	0
—	—	—	44	27	263	1.9	151	0	0.08	0.04	0.4	0
—	—	—	377	603	756	2.5	381	0	0.37	0.95	3.6	0
—	—	—	32	50	63	0.2	32	0	0.03	0.08	0.3	0
11.7	16.3	8.8	225	262	748	6.9	469	690	0.82	0.91	7.7	1
2.0	2.7	1.5	38	44	125	1.2	78	120	0.14	0.15	1.3	Trace
0.8	1.2	0.7	14	40	59	0.3	21	40	0.05	0.05	0.4	Trace
2.0	1.6	0.6	21	47	71	0.4	42	60	0.05	0.06	0.4	Trace
50.0	44.9	17.0	645	653	1,162	16.6	1,439	1,660	1.06	1.65	10.1	1
3.1	2.8	1.1	40	41	72	1.0	90	100	0.07	0.10	0.6	Trace
1.6	1.4	0.5	20	21	37	0.5	46	50	0.03	0.05	0.3	Trace
9.7	16.6	10.0	291	513	570	8.6	1,562	Trace	0.84	1.00	7.4	Trace
1.1	1.8	1.1	32	57	63	0.9	173	Trace	0.09	0.11	0.8	Trace

FOOD	Approximate Measures, Units, or Weight	Weight (g)	Water (%)	Food Energy (C)	Protein (g)	Fat (g)
White, 2-layer with chocolate icing:						
Whole cake (8- or 9-in. diam.)	1	1,140	21	4,000	44	122
Piece, 1/16 of cake	1	71	21	250	3	8
Yellow, 2-layer with chocolate icing:						
Whole cake (8- or 9-in. diam.)	1	1,108	26	3,735	45	125
Piece, 1/16 of cake	1	69	26	235	3	8
Cakes made from home recipes using enriched flour:[47]						
Boston cream pie with custard filling:						
Whole cake (8-in. diam.)	1	825	35	2,490	41	78
Piece, 1/12 of cake	1	69	35	210	3	6
Fruitcake, dark:						
Loaf, 1 lb (7½ × 2 × 1½ in.)	1 lb	454	18	1,720	22	69
Slice, 1/30 of loaf	1 slice	15	18	55	1	2
Plain, sheet cake:						
Without icing:						
Whole cake (9-in. square)	1	777	25	2,830	35	108
Piece, 1/9 of cake	1	86	25	315	4	12
With uncooked white icing:						
Whole cake (9-in. square)	1	1,096	21	4,020	37	129
Piece, 1/9 of cake	1	121	21	445	4	14
Pound cake:[49]						
Loaf, 8½ × 3½ × 3¼ in.	1	565	16	2,725	31	170
Slice, 1/17 of loaf	1	33	16	160	2	10
Sponge cake:						
Whole cake (9¾-in. diam. tube cake)	1	790	32	2,345	60	45
Piece, 1/12 of cake	1	66	32	195	5	4
Cookies made with enriched flour:[50][51]						
Brownie with nuts:						
Homemade, 1¾ × 1¾ × ⅞ in.:						
From home recipe	1	20	10	95	1	6
From commercial recipe	1	20	11	85	1	4
Frozen, with chocolate icing,[52] 1½ × 1¾ × ⅞ in.	1	25	13	105	1	5
Chocolate chip:						
Commercial, 2¼-in. diam., ⅜ in. thick	4	42	3	200	2	9
Homemade, 2⅓-in. diam.	4	40	3	205	2	12
Fig bars, square (1⅝ × 1⅝ × ⅜ in.) or rectangular (1½ × 1¾ × ½ in.)	4	56	14	200	2	3
Gingersnaps, 2-in. diam., ¼ in. thick	4	28	3	90	2	2
Macaroons, 2¾-in. diam., ¼ in. thick	2	38	4	180	2	9
Oatmeal with raisins, 2⅝-in. diam., ¼ in. thick	4	52	3	235	3	8
Plain, prepared from commercial chilled dough, 2½-in. diam., ¼ in. thick	4	48	5	240	2	12
Sandwich type (chocolate or vanilla), 1¾-in. diam., ⅜ in. thick	4	40	2	200	2	9
Vanilla wafers, 1¾-in. diam., ¼ in. thick	10	40	3	185	2	6

| | NUTRIENTS IN INDICATED QUANTITY | | | | | | | | | | | |
| FATTY ACIDS | | | | | | | | | | | | |
Saturated (Total) (g)	Unsaturated Oleic (g)	Unsaturated Linoleic (g)	Carbohydrate (g)	Calcium (mg)	Phosphorus (mg)	Iron (mg)	Potassium (mg)	Vitamin A Value (IU)	Vitamin B1 (mg)	Vitamin B2 (mg)	Niacin (mg)	Vitamin C (mg)
48.2	46.4	20.0	716	1,129	2,041	11.4	1,322	680	1.50	1.77	12.5	2
3.0	2.9	1.2	45	70	127	0.7	82	40	0.09	0.11	0.8	Trace
47.8	47.8	20.3	638	1,008	2,017	12.2	1,208	1,550	1.24	1.67	10.6	2
3.0	3.0	1.3	40	63	126	0.8	75	100	0.08	0.10	0.7	Trace
23.0	30.1	15.2	412	553	833	8.2	734[48]	1,730	1.04	1.27	9.6	2
1.9	2.5	1.3	34	46	70	0.7	61[48]	140	0.09	0.11	0.8	Trace
14.4	33.5	14.8	271	327	513	11.8	2,250	540	0.72	0.73	4.9	2
0.5	1.1	0.5	9	11	17	0.4	74	20	0.02	0.02	0.2	Trace
29.5	44.4	23.9	434	497	793	8.5	614[48]	1,320	1.21	1.40	10.2	2
3.3	4.9	2.6	48	55	88	0.9	68[48]	150	0.13	0.15	1.1	Trace
42.2	49.5	24.4	694	548	822	8.2	669[48]	2,190	1.22	1.47	10.2	2
4.7	5.5	2.7	77	61	91	0.8	74[48]	240	0.14	0.16	1.1	Trace
42.9	73.1	39.6	273	107	418	7.9	345	1,410	0.90	0.99	7.3	0
2.5	4.3	2.3	16	6	24	0.5	20	80	0.05	0.06	0.4	0
13.1	15.8	5.7	427	237	885	13.4	687	3,560	1.10	1.64	7.4	Trace
1.1	1.3	0.5	36	20	74	1.1	57	300	0.09	0.14	0.6	Trace
1.5	3.0	1.2	10	8	30	0.4	38	40	0.04	0.03	0.2	Trace
0.9	1.4	1.3	13	9	27	0.4	34	20	0.03	0.02	0.2	Trace
2.0	2.2	0.7	15	10	31	0.4	44	50	0.03	0.03	0.2	Trace
2.8	2.9	2.2	29	16	48	1.0	56	50	0.10	0.17	0.9	Trace
3.5	4.5	2.9	24	14	40	0.8	47	40	0.06	0.06	0.5	Trace
0.8	1.2	0.7	42	44	34	1.0	111	60	0.04	0.14	0.9	Trace
0.7	1.0	0.6	22	20	13	0.7	129	20	0.08	0.06	0.7	0
—	—	—	25	10	32	0.3	176	0	0.02	0.06	0.2	0
2.0	3.3	2.0	38	11	53	1.4	192	30	0.15	0.10	1.0	Trace
3.0	5.2	2.9	31	17	35	0.6	23	30	0.10	0.08	0.9	0
2.2	3.9	2.2	28	10	96	0.7	15	0	0.06	0.10	0.7	0
—	—	—	30	16	25	0.6	29	50	0.10	0.09	0.8	0

FOOD	Approximate Measures. Units. or Weight	Weight (g)	Water (%)	Food Energy (C)	Protein (g)	Fat (g)
Cornmeal:						
Whole-grain, unbolted, dry form	1 c	122	12	435	11	5
Bolted (nearly whole grain), dry form	1 c	122	12	440	11	4
Degermed, enriched:						
Dry form	1 c	138	12	500	11	2
Cooked	1 c	240	88	120	3	Trace
Degermed, unenriched:						
Dry form	1 c	138	12	500	11	2
Cooked	1 c	240	88	120	3	Trace
Crackers:[38]						
Graham, plain, 2½-in. square	2	14	6	55	1	1
Rye wafers, whole grain, 1⅞ × 3½ in.	2	13	6	45	2	Trace
Saltines, made with enriched flour	4 crackers	11	4	50	1	1
Danish pastry (enriched flour), plain without fruit or nuts:[54]						
Ounce	1 ox	28	22	120	2	7
Packaged ring, 12 oz	1	340	22	1,435	25	80
Round piece, about 4¼-in. diam. × 1 in.	1 pastry	65	22	275	5	15
Doughnut, made with enriched flour:[38]						
Cake type, plain, 2½-in. diam., 1 in. high	1	25	24	100	1	5
Yeast-leavened, glazed, 3¾-in. diam., 1¼ in. high	1	50	26	205	3	11
Macaroni, enriched, cooked (cut lengths, elbows, shells):						
Firm stage (hot)	1 c	130	64	190	7	1
Tender stage:						
Cold	1 c	105	73	115	4	Trace
Hot	1 c	140	73	155	5	1
Macaroni (enriched) and cheese:						
Canned[55]	1 c	240	80	230	9	10
Homemade (served hot)[56]	1 c	200	38	430	17	22
Muffin made with enriched flour:[38]						
Homemade:						
Blueberry, 2⅜-in. diam., 1½-in. high	1	40	39	110	3	4
Bran	1	40	35	105	3	4
Corn (enriched, degermed cornmeal and flour), 2⅜-in. diam., 1½ in. high	1	40	33	125	3	4
Plain, 3-in. diam., 1½ in. high	1	40	38	120	3	4
From mix, egg, milk:						
Corn, 2⅜-in. diam., 1½ in. high[58]	1	40	30	130	3	4
Noodles, chow mein, canned	1 c	45	1	220	6	11
Noodles (egg noodles), enriched, cooked	1 c	160	71	200	7	.2
Pancakes, (4-in. diam.):[38]						
Buckwheat, made from mix (with buckwheat and enriched flours), egg and milk added	1 cake	27	58	55	2	2

Saturated (Total) (g)	Oleic (g)	Linoleic (g)	Carbohydrate (g)	Calcium (mg)	Phosphorus (mg)	Iron (mg)	Potassium (mg)	Vitamin A Value (IU)	Vitamin B1 (mg)	Vitamin B2 (mg)	Niacin (mg)	Vitamin C (mg)
0.5	1.0	2.5	90	24	312	2.9	346	620[53]	0.46	0.13	2.4	0
0.5	0.9	2.1	91	21	272	2.2	303	590[53]	0.37	0.10	2.3	0
0.2	0.4	0.9	108	8	137	4.0	166	610[53]	0.61	0.36	4.8	0
Trace	0.1	0.2	26	2	34	1.0	38	140[53]	0.14	0.10	1.2	0
0.2	0.4	0.9	108	8	137	1.5	166	610[53]	0.19	0.07	1.4	0
Trace	0.1	0.2	26	2	34	0.5	38	140[53]	0.05	0.02	0.2	0
0.3	0.5	0.3	10	6	21	0.5	55	0	0.02	0.08	0.5	0
—	—	—	10	7	50	0.5	78	0	0.04	0.03	0.2	0
0.3	0.5	0.4	8	2	10	0.5	13	0	0.05	0.05	0.4	0
2.0	2.7	1.4	13	14	31	0.5	32	90	0.08	0.08	0.7	Trace
24.3	31.7	16.5	155	170	371	6.1	381	1,050	0.97	1.01	8.6	Trace
4.7	6.1	3.2	30	33	71	1.2	73	200	0.18	0.19	1.7	Trace
1.2	2.0	1.1	13	10	48	0.4	23	20	0.05	0.05	0.4	Trace
3.3	5.8	3.3	22	16	33	0.6	34	25	0.10	0.10	0.8	0
—	—	—	39	14	85	1.4	103	0	0.23	0.13	1.8	0
—	—	—	24	8	53	0.9	64	0	0.15	0.08	1.2	0
—	—	—	32	11	70	1.3	85	0	0.20	0.11	1.5	0
4.2	3.1	1.4	26	199	182	1.0	139	260	0.12	0.24	1.0	Trace
8.9	8.8	2.9	40	362	322	1.8	240	860	0.20	0.40	1.8	Trace
1.1	1.4	0.7	17	34	53	0.6	46	90	0.09	0.10	0.7	Trace
1.2	1.4	0.8	17	57	162	1.5	172	90	0.07	0.10	1.7	Trace
1.2	1.6	0.9	19	42	68	0.7	54	120[57]	0.10	0.10	0.7	Trace
1.0	1.7	1.0	17	42	60	0.6	50	40	0.09	0.12	0.9	Trace
1.2	1.7	0.9	20	96	152	0.6	44	100[57]	0.08	0.09	0.7	Trace
—	—	—	26	—	—	—	—	—	—	—	—	—
—	—	—	37	16	94	1.4	70	110	0.22	0.13	1.9	0
0.8	0.9	0.4	6	59	91	0.4	66	60	0.04	0.05	0.2	Trace

FOOD	Approximate Measures, Units, or Weight	Weight (g)	Water (%)	Food Energy (C)	Protein (g)	Fat (g)
Plain:						
Homemade with enriched flour	1 cake	27	50	60	2	2
Made from mix with enriched flour; egg and milk added	1 cake	77	51	60	2	2
Pies, piecrust made with enriched flour and vegetable shortening (9-in. diam.):						
Apple:						
Whole	1 pie	945	48	2,420	21	105
Sector, 1/7 of pie	1 sector	135	48	345	3	15
Banana cream:						
Whole	1 pie	910	54	2,010	41	85
Sector, 1/7 of pie	1 sector	130	54	285	6	12
Blueberry:						
Whole	1 pie	945	51	2,285	23	102
Sector, 1/7 of pie	1 sector	135	51	325	3	15
Cherry:						
Whole	1 pie	945	47	2,465	25	107
Sector, 1/7 of pie	1 sector	135	47	350	4	15
Custard:						
Whole	1 pie	910	58	1,985	56	101
Sector, 1/7 of pie	1 sector	130	58	285	8	14
Lemon meringue:						
Whole	1 pie	840	47	2,140	31	86
Sector, 1/7 of pie	1 sector	120	47	305	4	12
Mince:						
Whole	1 pie	945	43	2,560	24	109
Sector, 1/7 of pie	1 sector	135	43	365	3	16
Peach:						
Whole	1 pie	945	48	2,410	24	101
Sector, 1/7 of pie	1 sector	135	48	345	3	14
Pecan:						
Whole	1 pie	825	20	3,450	42	189
Sector, 1/7 of pie	1 sector	118	20	495	6	27
Pumpkin:						
Whole	1 pie	910	59	1,920	36	102
Sector, 1/7 of pie	1 sector	130	59	275	5	15
Piecrust (homemade) made with enriched flour and vegetable shortening, baked, 9-in. diam.	1 shell	180	15	900	11	60
Piecrust mix with enriched flour and vegetable shortening, 10-oz. package prepared and baked, 9-in. diam.	1 shell (2-crust pie)	320	10	1,485	20	93
Pizza (cheese) baked, 4¾-in. sector; 1/8 of 12-in.-diam pie[19]	1 sector	60	45	145	6	4

NUTRIENTS IN INDICATED QUANTITY

Saturated (Total) (g)	Oleic (g)	Linoleic (g)	Carbohydrate (g)	Calcium (mg)	Phosphorus (mg)	Iron (mg)	Potassium (mg)	Vitamin A Value (IU)	Vitamin B1 (mg)	Vitamin B2 (mg)	Niacin (mg)	Vitamin C (mg)
0.5	0.8	0.5	9	27	38	0.4	33	30	0.06	0.07	0.5	Trace
0.7	0.7	0.3	9	58	70	0.3	42	70	0.04	0.06	0.2	Trace
27.0	44.5	25.2	360	76	208	6.6	756	280	1.06	0.79	9.3	9
3.9	6.4	3.6	51	11	30	0.9	108	40	0.15	0.11	1.3	2
26.7	33.2	16.2	279	601	746	7.3	1,847	2,280	0.77	1.51	7.0	9
3.8	4.7	2.3	40	86	107	1.0	264	330	0.11	0.22	1.0	1
24.8	43.7	25.1	330	104	217	9.5	614	280	1.03	0.80	10.0	28
3.5	6.2	3.6	47	15	31	1.4	88	40	0.15	0.11	1.4	4
28.2	45.0	25.3	363	132	236	6.6	992	4,160	1.09	0.84	9.8	Trace
4.0	6.4	3.6	52	19	34	0.9	142	590	0.16	0.12	1.4	Trace
33.9	38.5	17.5	213	874	1,028	8.2	1,247	2,090	0.79	1.92	5.6	0
4.8	5.5	2.5	30	125	147	1.2	178	300	0.11	0.27	0.8	0
26.1	33.8	16.4	317	118	412	6.7	420	1,430	0.61	0.84	5.2	25
3.7	4.8	2.3	45	17	59	1.0	60	200	0.09	0.12	0.7	4
28.0	45.9	25.2	389	265	359	13.3	1,682	20	0.96	0.86	9.8	9
4.0	6.6	3.6	56	38	51	1.9	240	Trace	0.14	0.12	1.4	1
24.8	43.7	25.1	361	95	274	8.5	1,408	6,900	1.04	0.97	14.0	28
3.5	6.2	3.6	52	14	39	1.2	201	990	0.15	0.14	2.0	4
27.8	101.0	44.2	423	388	850	25.6	1,015	1,320	1.80	0.95	6.9	Trace
4.0	14.4	6.3	61	55	122	3.7	145	190	0.26	0.14	1.0	Trace
37.4	37.5	16.6	223	464	628	7.3	1,456	22,480	0.78	1.27	7.0	Trace
5.4	5.4	2.4	32	66	90	1.0	208	3,210	0.11	0.18	1.0	Trace
14.8	26.1	14.9	79	25	90	3.1	89	0	0.47	0.40	5.0	0
22.7	39.7	23.4	141	131	272	6.1	179	0	1.07	0.79	9.9	0
1.7	1.5	0.6	22	86	89	1.1	67	230	0.16	0.18	1.6	4

FOOD	Approximate Measures, Units, or Weight	Weight (g)	Water (%)	Food Energy (C)	Protein (g)	Fat (g)
Popcorn, popped:						
Plain, large kernel	1 c	6	4	25	1	Trace
With oil (coconut) and salt added, large kernel	1 c	9	3	40	1	2
Sugar coated	1 c	35	4	135	2	1
Pretzels, made with enriched flour:						
Dutch, twisted, 2¾ × 2⅝ in.	1	16	5	60	2	1
Thin, twisted, 3¼ × 2¼ × ¼ in.	10	60	5	235	6	3
Stick, 2¼ in. long	10	3	5	10	Trace	Trace
Rice, white, enriched:						
Instant, ready-to-serve, hot	1 c	165	73	180	4	Trace
Long grain:						
Raw	1 c	185	12	670	12	1
Cooked, served hot	1 c	205	73	225	4	Trace
Parboiled:						
Raw	1 c	185	10	685	14	1
Cooked, served hot	1 c	175	73	185	4	Trace
Roll, enriched:[38]						
Commercial:						
Brown-and-serve (1 oz), browned	1	26	27	85	2	2
Cloverleaf or pan, 2½-in. diam., 2 in. high	1	28	31	85	2	2
Frankfurter and hamburger (8 per 11½-oz package)	1	40	31	120	3	2
Hard, 3¾-in. diam., 2 in. high	1	50	25	155	5	2
Hoagie or submarine, 11½ × 3 × 2½ in.	1	135	31	390	12	4
Homemade:						
Cloverleaf, 2½-in. diam., 2 in. high	1	35	26	120	3	3
Spaghetti, enriched, cooked:						
Firm stage, al dente, served hot	1 c	130	64	190	7	1
Tender stage, served hot	1 c	140	73	155	5	1
Spaghetti (enriched) in tomato sauce with cheese:						
Canned	1 c	250	80	190	6	2
Homemade	1 c	250	77	260	9	9
Spaghetti (enriched) with meatballs and tomato sauce:						
Canned	1 c	250	78	260	12	10
Homemade	1 c	248	70	330	19	12
Toaster pastry	1	50	12	200	3	6
Waffles, made with enriched flour, 7-in. diam.:[38]						
Homemade	1	75	41	210	7	7
From mix, egg and milk added	1	75	42	205	7	8

Saturated (Total) (g)	Oleic (g)	Linoleic (g)	Carbohydrate (g)	Calcium (mg)	Phosphorus (mg)	Iron (mg)	Potassium (mg)	Vitamin A Value (IU)	Vitamin B1 (mg)	Vitamin B2 (mg)	Niacin (mg)	Vitamin C (mg)
Trace	0.1	0.2	5	1	17	0.2	—	—	—	0.01	0.1	0
1.5	0.2	0.2	5	1	19	0.2	—	—	—	0.01	0.2	0
0.5	0.2	0.4	30	2	47	0.5	—	—	—	0.02	0.4	0
—	—	—	12	4	21	0.2	21	0	0.05	0.04	0.7	0
—	—	—	46	13	79	0.9	78	0	0.20	0.15	2.5	0
—	—	—	2	1	4	Trace	4	0	0.01	0.01	0.1	0
Trace	Trace	Trace	40	5	31	1.3	—	0	0.21	59	1.7	0
0.2	0.2	0.2	149	44	174	5.4	170	0	0.81	0.06	6.5	0
0.1	0.1	0.1	50	21	57	1.8	57	0	0.23	0.02	2.1	0
0.2	0.1	0.2	150	111	370	5.4	278	0	0.81	0.07	6.5	0
0.1	0.1	0.1	41	33	100	1.4	75	0	0.19	0.02	2.1	0
0.4	0.7	0.5	14	20	23	0.5	25	Trace	0.10	0.06	0.9	Trace
0.4	0.6	0.4	15	21	24	0.5	27	Trace	0.11	0.07	0.9	Trace
0.5	0.8	0.6	21	30	34	0.8	38	Trace	0.16	0.10	1.3	Trace
0.4	0.6	0.5	30	24	46	1.2	49	Trace	0.20	0.12	1.7	Trace
0.9	1.4	1.4	75	58	115	3.0	122	Trace	0.54	0.32	4.5	Trace
0.8	1.1	0.7	20	16	36	0.7	41	30	0.12	0.12	1.2	Trace
—	—	—	39	14	85	1.4	103	0	0.23	0.13	1.8	0
—	—	—	32	11	70	1.3	85	0	0.20	0.11	1.5	0
0.5	0.3	0.4	39	40	88	2.8	303	930	0.35	0.28	4.5	10
2.0	5.4	0.7	37	80	135	2.3	408	1,080	0.25	0.18	2.3	13
2.2	3.3	3.9	29	53	113	3.3	245	1,000	0.15	0.18	2.3	5
3.3	6.3	0.9	39	124	236	3.7	665	1,590	0.25	0.30	4.0	22
—	—	—	36	54[60]	67[60]	1.9	74[60]	500	0.16	0.17	2.1	60
2.3	2.8	1.4	28	85	130	1.3	109	250	0.17	0.23	1.4	Trace
2.8	2.9	1.2	27	179	257	1.0	146	170	0.14	0.22	0.9	Trace

FOOD	Approximate Measures, Units, or Weight	Weight (g)	Water (%)	Food Energy (C)	Protein (g)	Fat (g)
Wheat flour:						
All-purpose or family flour, enriched:						
Sifted, spooned	1 c	115	12	420	12	1
Unsifted, spooned	1 c	125	12	455	13	1
Cake or pastry flour, enriched, sifted, spooned	1 c	96	12	350	7	1
Self-rising, enriched, unsifted, spooned	1 c	125	12	440	12	1
Whole wheat, from hard wheats, stirred	1 c	120	12	400	16	2
Legumes (dry), nuts, seeds; related products						
Almonds, shelled:						
Chopped (about 130 almonds)	1 c	130	5	775	24	70
Slivered, not pressed down (about 115 almonds)	1 c	115	5	690	21	62
Beans, dry:						
Common varieties as Great Northern, navy, and others:						
Canned, solids and liquid:						
White with—						
Frankfurters (sliced)	1 c	255	71	365	19	18
Pork and sweet sauce	1 c	255	66	385	16	12
Pork and tomato sauce	1 c	255	71	310	16	7
Red kidney	1 c	255	76	230	15	1
Cooked, drained:						
Great Northern	1 c	180	69	210	14	1
Pea (navy)	1 c	190	69	225	15	1
Lima, cooked, drained	1 c	190	64	260	16	1
Black-eyed peas, dry, cooked (with residual cooking liquid)	1 c	250	80	190	13	1
Brazil nuts, shelled (6–8 large kernels)	1 oz	28	5	185	4	19
Cashew nuts, roasted in oil	1 c	140	5	785	24	64
Coconut meat, fresh:						
Piece, about 2 × 2 × ½ in.	1	45	51	155	2	16
Shredded or grated, not pressed down	1 c	80	51	275	3	28
Filberts (hazelnuts), chopped (about 80 kernels)	1 c	115	6	730	14	72
Lentils, whole, cooked	1 c	200	72	210	16	Trace
Peanuts, roasted in oil, salted (whole, halves, chopped)	1 c	144	2	840	37	72
Peanut butter	1 T	16	2	95	4	8
Peas, split, dry, cooked	1 c	200	70	230	16	1
Pecans, chopped or pieces (about 120 large halves)	1 c	118	3	810	11	84
Pumpkin and squash kernels, dry, hulled	1 c	140	4	775	41	65
Sunflower seeds, dry, hulled	1 c	145	5	810	35	69
Walnuts:						
Black:						
Chopped or broken kernels	1 c	125	3	785	26	74
Ground (finely)	1 c	80	3	500	16	47

NUTRIENTS IN INDICATED QUANTITY

Saturated (Total) (g)	Oleic (g)	Linoleic (g)	Carbohydrate (g)	Calcium (mg)	Phosphorus (mg)	Iron (mg)	Potassium (mg)	Vitamin A Value (IU)	Vitamin B1 (mg)	Vitamin B2 (mg)	Niacin (mg)	Vitamin C (mg)
0.2	0.1	0.5	88	18	100	3.3	109	0	0.74	0.46	6.1	0
0.2	0.1	0.5	95	20	109	3.6	119	0	0.80	0.50	6.6	0
0.1	0.1	0.3	76	16	70	2.8	91	0	0.61	0.38	5.1	0
0.2	0.1	0.5	93	331	583	3.6	—	0	0.80	0.50	6.6	0
0.4	0.2	1.0	85	49	446	4.0	444	0	0.66	0.14	5.2	0
5.6	47.7	12.8	25	304	655	6.1	1,005	0	0.31	1.20	4.6	Trace
5.0	42.2	11.3	22	269	580	5.4	889	0	0.28	1.06	4.0	Trace
—	—	—	32	94	303	4.8	668	330	0.18	0.15	3.3	Trace
4.3	5.0	1.1	54	161	291	5.9	—	—	0.15	0.10	1.3	—
2.4	2.8	0.6	48	138	235	4.6	536	330	0.20	0.08	1.5	5
—	—	—	42	74	278	4.6	673	10	0.13	0.10	1.5	—
—	—	—	38	90	266	4.9	749	0	0.25	0.13	1.3	0
—	—	—	40	95	281	5.1	790	0	0.27	0.13	1.3	0
—	—	—	49	55	293	5.9	1,163	—	0.25	0.11	1.3	—
—	—	—	35	43	238	3.3	573	30	0.40	0.10	1.0	—
4.8	6.2	7.1	3	53	196	1.0	203	Trace	0.27	0.03	0.5	—
12.9	36.8	10.2	41	53	522	5.3	650	140	0.60	0.35	2.5	—
14.0	0.9	0.3	4	6	43	0.8	115	0	0.02	0.01	0.2	1
24.8	1.6	0.5	8	10	76	1.4	205	0	0.04	0.02	0.4	2
5.1	55.2	7.3	19	240	388	3.9	810	—	0.53	—	1.0	Trace
—	—	—	39	50	238	4.2	498	40	0.14	0.12	1.2	0
13.7	33.0	20.7	27	107	577	3.0	971	—	0.46	0.19	24.8	0
1.5	3.7	2.3	3	9	61	0.3	100	—	0.02	0.02	2.4	0
—	—	—	42	22	178	3.4	592	80	0.30	0.18	1.8	—
7.2	50.5	20.0	17	86	341	2.8	712	150	1.01	0.15	1.1	2
11.8	23.5	27.5	21	71	1,602	15.7	1,386	100	0.34	0.27	3.4	—
8.2	13.7	43.2	29	174	1,214	10.3	1,334	70	2.84	0.33	78	—
6.3	13.3	45.7	19	Trace	713	7.5	575	380	0.28	0.14	0.9	—
4.0	8.5	29.2	12	Trace	456	4.8	368	240	0.18	0.09	0.6	—

FOOD	Approximate Measures. Units. or Weight	Weight (g)	Water (%)	Food Energy (C)	Protein (g)	Fat (g)
Persian or English,						
Chopped (about 60 halves)	1 c	120	4	780	18	77
Sugars and sweets						
Cake icings:						
Boiled, white:						
Plain	1 c	94	18	295	1	0
With coconut	1 c	166	15	605	3	13
Uncooked:						
Chocolate made with milk and butter	1 c	275	14	1,035	9	38
Creamy fudge from mix and water	1 c	245	15	830	7	16
White	1 c	319	11	1,200	2	21
Candy:						
Caramels, plain or chocolate	1 oz	28	8	115	1	3
Chocolate:						
Milk, plain	1 oz	28	1	145	2	9
Semisweet, small pieces (60 per ounce)	1 c or 6 oz	170	1	860	7	61
Chocolate-covered peanuts	1 oz	28	1	160	5	12
Fondant, uncoated (mints, candy corn, other)	1 oz	28	8	105	Trace	1
Fudge, chocolate, plain	1 oz	28	8	115	1	3
Gumdrops	1 oz	28	12	100	Trace	Trace
Hard	1 oz	28	1	110	0	Trace
Marshmallows	1 oz	28	17	90	1	Trace
Chocolate-flavored beverage powders (about 4 heaping teaspoons per ounce):						
With nonfat milk	1 oz	28	2	100	5	1
Without milk	1 oz	28	1	100	1	1
Honey, strained or extracted	1 T	21	17	65	Trace	0
James and preserves	1 T	20	29	55	Trace	Trace
	1 packet	14	29	40	Trace	Trace
Jellies	1 T	18	29	50	Trace	Trace
	1 packet	14	29	40	Trace	Trace
Syrups:						
Chocolate-flavored syrup or topping:						
Fudge type	1 fl oz or 2 T	38	25	125	2	5
Thin type	1 fl oz or 2 T	38	32	90	1	1
Molasses, cane:						
Light (first extraction)	1 T	20	24	50	—	—
Blackstrap (third extraction)	1 T	20	24	45	—	—
Sorghum	1 T	21	23	55	—	—
Table blends, chiefly corn, light and dark	1 T	21	24	60	0	0
Sugar:						
Brown, pressed down	1 c	220	2	820	0	0
White:						
Granulated	1 c	200	1	770	0	0
	1 T	12	1	45	0	0
	1 packet	6	1	23	0	0
Powdered, sifted, spooned into cup	1 c	100	1	385	0	0

NUTRIENTS IN INDICATED QUANTITY

| FATTY ACIDS | | | | | | | | | | | | |
Saturated (Total) (g)	Unsaturated Oleic (g)	Unsaturated Linoleic (g)	Carbohydrate (g)	Calcium (mg)	Phosphorus (mg)	Iron (mg)	Potassium (mg)	Vitamin A value (IU)	Vitamin B1 (mg)	Vitamin B2 (mg)	Niacin (mg)	Vitamin C (mg)
8.4	11.8	42.2	19	119	456	3.7	540	40	0.40	0.16	1.1	2
0	0	0	75	2	2	Trace	17	0	Trace	0.03	Trace	0
11.0	0.9	Trace	124	10	50	0.8	277	0	0.02	0.07	0.3	0
23.4	11.7	1.0	185	165	305	3.3	536	580	0.06	0.28	0.6	1
5.1	6.7	3.1	183	96	218	2.7	238	Trace	0.05	0.20	0.7	Trace
12.7	5.1	0.5	260	48	38	Trace	57	860	Trace	0.06	Trace	Trace
1.6	1.1	0.1	22	42	35	0.4	54	Trace	0.01	0.05	0.1	Trace
5.5	3.0	0.3	16	65	65	0.3	109	80	0.02	0.10	0.1	Trace
36.2	19.8	1.7	97	51	255	4.4	553	30	0.02	0.14	0.9	0
4.0	4.7	2.1	11	33	84	0.4	143	Trace	0.10	0.05	2.1	Trace
0.1	0.3	0.1	25	4	2	0.3	1	0	Trace	Trace	Trace	0
1.3	1.4	0.6	21	22	24	0.3	42	Trace	0.01	0.03	0.1	Trace
—	—	—	25	2	Trace	0.1	1	0	0	Trace	Trace	0
—	—	—	28	6	2	0.5	1	0	0	0	0	0
—	—	—	23	5	2	0.5	2	0	0	Trace	Trace	0
0.5	0.3	Trace	20	167	155	0.5	227	10	0.04	0.21	0.2	1
0.4	0.2	Trace	25	9	48	0.6	142	—	0.01	0.03	0.1	0
0	0	0	17	1	1	0.1	11	0	Trace	0.01	0.1	Trace
—	—	—	14	4	2	0.2	18	Trace	Trace	0.01	Trace	Trace
—	—	—	10	3	1	0.1	12	Trace	Trace	Trace	Trace	Trace
—	—	—	13	4	1	0.3	14	Trace	Trace	0.01	Trace	1
—	—	—	10	3	1	0.2	11	Trace	Trace	Trace	Trace	1
3.1	1.6	0.1	20	48	60	0.5	107	60	0.02	0.08	0.2	Trace
0.5	0.3	Trace	24	6	35	0.6	106	Trace	0.01	0.03	0.2	0
—	—	—	13	33	9	0.9	183	—	0.01	0.01	Trace	—
—	—	—	11	137	17	3.2	585	—	0.02	0.04	0.4	—
0	—	—	14	35	5	2.6	—	—	—	0.02	Trace	—
0	0	0	15	9	3	0.8	1	0	0	0	0	0
0	0	0	212	187	42	7.5	757	0	0.02	0.07	0.4	0
0	0	0	199	0	0	0.2	6	0	0	0	0	0
0	0	0	12	0	0	Trace	Trace	0	0	0	0	0
0	0	0	6	0	0	Trace	Trace	0	0	0	0	0
0	0	0	100	0	0	0.1	3	0	0	0	0	0

Vegetables and vegetable products

FOOD	Approximate Measures, Units, or Weight	Weight (g)	Water (%)	Food Energy (C)	Protein (g)	Fat (g)
Vegetables and vegetable products						
Asparagus, green:						
Cooked, drained:						
Cuts and tips, 1½- to 2-in. lengths:						
From raw	1 c	145	94	30	3	Trace
From frozen	1 c	180	93	40	6	Trace
Spears, ½-in. diam. at base:						
From raw	4	60	94	10	1	Trace
From frozen	4	60	92	15	2	Trace
Canned, spears, ½-in. diam. at base	4	80	93	15	2	Trace
Beans:						
Lima, immature seeds, frozen, cooked, drained:						
Thick-seeded types (Fordhooks)	1 c	170	74	170	10	Trace
Thin-seeded types (baby limas)	1 c	180	69	210	13	Trace
Snap:						
Green:						
Canned, drained solids (cuts)	1 c	135	92	30	2	Trace
Cooked, drained:						
From raw (cuts and French style)	1 c	125	92	30	2	Trace
From frozen:						
Cuts	1 c	135	92	35	2	Trace
French style	1 c	130	92	35	2	Trace
Yellow or wax:						
Cooked, drained:						
From raw (cuts and French style)	1 c	125	93	30	2	Trace
From frozen (cuts)	1 c	135	92	35	2	Trace
Canned, drained solids (cuts)	1 c	135	92	30	2	Trace
Beans, mature. See Beans, dry, and Black-eyed peas, dry.						
Bean sprouts (mung):						
Raw	1 c	105	89	35	4	Trace
Cooked, drained	1 c	125	91	35	4	Trace
Beets:						
Canned, drained, solids:						
Whole, small	1 c	160	89	60	2	Trace
Diced or sliced	1 c	170	89	65	2	Trace
Cooked, drained, peeled:						
Whole, 2-in. diam.	2	100	91	30	1	Trace
Diced or sliced	1 c	170	91	55	1	Trace
Beet greens, leaves and stems, cooked, drained	1 c	145	94	25	2	Trace
Black-eyed peas, immature seeds, cooked and drained:						
From raw	1 c	165	72	180	13	1
From frozen	1 c	170	66	220	15	1

352

| FATTY ACIDS | | | Carbohydrate (g) | Calcium (mg) | Phosphorus (mg) | Iron (mg) | Potassium (mg) | Vitamin A Value (IU) | Vitamin B1 (mg) | Vitamin B2 (mg) | Niacin (mg) | Vitamin C (mg) |
Saturated (Total) (g)	Unsaturated Oleic (g)	Unsaturated Linoleic (g)										
—	—	—	5	30	73	0.9	265	1,310	0.23	0.26	2.0	38
—	—	—	6	40	115	2.2	396	1,530	0.25	0.23	1.8	41
—	—	—	2	13	30	0.4	110	540	0.10	0.11	0.8	16
—	—	—	2	13	40	0.7	143	470	0.10	0.08	0.7	16
—	—	—	3	15	42	1.5	133	640	0.05	0.08	0.6	12
—	—	—	32	34	153	2.9	724	390	0.12	0.09	1.7	29
—	—	—	40	63	227	4.7	709	400	0.16	0.09	2.2	22
—	—	—	7	61	34	2.0	128	630	0.04	0.07	0.4	5
—	—	—	7	63	46	0.8	189	680	0.09	0.11	0.4	15
—	—	—	8	54	43	0.9	205	780	0.09	0.12	0.5	7
—	—	—	8	49	39	1.2	177	690	0.08	0.10	0.4	9
—	—	—	6	63	46	0.8	189	290	0.09	0.11	0.6	16
—	—	—	8	47	42	0.9	221	140	0.09	0.11	0.5	8
—	—	—	7	61	34	2.0	128	140	0.04	0.07	0.4	7
—	—	—	7	20	67	1.4	234	20	0.14	0.14	0.8	20
—	—	—	7	21	60	1.1	195	30	0.11	0.13	0.9	8
—	—	—	14	30	29	1.1	267	30	0.02	0.05	0.2	5
—	—	—	15	32	31	1.2	284	30	0.02	0.05	0.2	5
—	—	—	7	14	23	0.5	208	20	0.03	0.04	0.3	6
—	—	—	12	24	39	0.9	354	30	0.05	0.07	0.5	10
—	—	—	5	144	36	2.8	481	7,400	0.10	0.22	0.4	22
—	—	—	30	40	241	3.5	625	580	0.50	0.18	2.3	28
—	—	—	40	43	286	4.8	573	290	0.68	0.19	2.4	15

FOOD	Approximate Measures, Units, or Weight	Weight (g)	Water (%)	Food Energy (C)	Protein (g)	Fat (g)
Broccoli, cooked, drained:						
From raw:						
Stalk, medium size	1	180	91	45	6	1
Stalks cut into 1/2-in. pieces	1 c	155	91	40	5	Trace
From frozen:						
Chopped	1 c	185	92	50	5	1
Stalk, 4 1/2 to 5 in. long	1	30	91	10	1	Trace
Brussels sprouts, cooked, drained:						
From raw, 7–8 sprouts (1 1/4- to 1 1/2-in. diam.)	1 c	155	88	55	7	1
From frozen	1 c	155	89	50	5	Trace
Cabbage:						
Common varieties:						
Raw:						
Coarsely shredded or sliced	1 c	70	92	15	1	Trace
Finely shredded or chopped	1 c	90	92	20	1	Trace
Cooked, drained	1 c	145	94	30	2	Trace
Red, raw, coarsely shredded or sliced	1 c	70	90	20	1	Trace
Savoy, raw, coarsely shredded or sliced	1 c	70	92	15	2	Trace
Cabbage, celery (also called pe-tsai or wongbok), raw, 1-in. pieces	1 c	75	95	10	1	Trace
Cabbage, white mustard (also called bok choy or pak choy), cooked, drained	1 c	170	05	25	2	Trace
Carrots:						
Raw, without crowns and tips, scraped:						
Grated	1 c	110	88	45	1	Trace
Whole, 7 1/2 by 1 1/8 in. or strips, 2 1/2 to 3 in. long	1 carrot or 18 strips	72	88	30	1	Trace
Canned:						
Sliced, drained solids	1 c	155	91	45	1	Trace
Strained or junior (baby food)	1 oz (1 3/4 to 2 T)	28	92	10	Trace	Trace
Cooked (crosswise cuts), drained	1 c	155	91	50	1	Trace
Cauliflower:						
Raw, chopped	1 c	115	91	31	3	Trace
Cooked, drained:						
From raw (flower buds)	1 c	125	93	30	3	Trace
From frozen (flowerets)	1 c	180	94	30	3	Trace
Celery, Pascal type, raw:						
Pieces, diced	1 c	120	94	20	1	Trace
Stalk, large outer, 8 by 1 1/2 in. at root end	1	40	94	5	Trace	Trace
Collards, cooked, drained:						
From raw (leaves without stems)	1 c	190	90	65	7	1
From frozen (chopped)	1 c	170	90	50	5	1
Corn, sweet:						
Cooked, drained:						
From raw, ear, 5 by 1 3/4 in.	1	140[61]	74	70	2	1

NUTRIENTS IN INDICATED QUANTITY

Saturated (Total) (g)	Oleic (g)	Linoleic (g)	Carbohydrate (g)	Calcium (mg)	Phosphorus (mg)	Iron (mg)	Potassium (mg)	Vitamin A Value (IU)	Vitamin B1 (mg)	Vitamin B2 (mg)	Niacin (mg)	Vitamin C (mg)
—	—	—	8	158	112	1.4	481	4,500	0.16	0.36	1.4	162
—	—	—	7	136	96	1.2	414	3,880	0.14	0.31	1.2	140
—	—	—	9	100	104	1.3	392	4,810	0.11	0.22	0.9	105
—	—	—	1	12	17	0.2	66	570	0.02	0.03	0.2	22
—	—	—	10	50	112	1.7	423	810	0.12	0.22	1.2	135
—	—	—	10	33	95	1.2	457	880	0.12	0.16	0.9	126
—	—	—	4	34	20	0.3	163	90	0.04	0.04	0.2	33
—	—	—	5	44	26	0.4	210	120	0.05	0.05	0.3	42
—	—	—	6	64	29	0.4	236	190	0.06	0.06	0.4	48
—	—	—	5	29	25	0.6	188	30	0.06	0.04	0.3	43
—	—	—	3	47	38	0.6	188	140	0.04	0.06	0.2	39
—	—	—	2	32	30	0.5	190	110	0.04	0.03	0.5	19
—	—	—	4	252	56	1.0	364	5,270	0.07	0.14	1.2	26
—	—	—	11	41	40	0.8	375	12,100	0.07	0.06	0.7	9
—	—	—	7	27	26	0.5	246	7,930	0.04	0.04	0.4	6
—	—	—	10	47	34	1.1	186	23,250	0.03	0.05	0.6	3
—	—	—	2	7	6	0.1	51	3,690	0.01	0.01	0.1	1
—	—	—	11	51	48	0.9	344	16,280	0.08	0.08	0.8	9
—	—	—	6	29	64	1.3	339	70	0.13	0.12	0.8	90
—	—	—	5	26	53	0.9	258	80	0.11	0.10	0.8	69
—	—	—	6	31	68	0.9	373	50	0.07	0.09	0.7	74
—	—	—	5	47	34	0.4	409	320	0.04	0.04	0.4	11
—	—	—	2	16	11	0.1	136	110	0.01	0.01	0.1	4
—	—	—	10	357	99	1.5	498	14,820	0.21	0.38	2.3	144
—	—	—	10	299	87	1.7	401	11,560	0.10	0.24	1.0	56
—	—	—	16	2	69	0.5	151	310[62]	0.09	0.08	1.1	7

FOOD	Approximate Measures, Units, or Weight	Weight (g)	Water (%)	Food Energy (C)	Protein (g)	Fat (g)
From frozen:						
Ear, 5 in. long	1	229[61]	73	120	4	1
Kernels	1 c	165	77	130	5	1
Canned:						
Cream style	1 c	256	76	210	5	2
Whole kernel:						
Vacuum pack	1 c	210	76	175	5	1
Wet pack, drained solids	1 c	165	76	140	4	1
Cowpeas. See Black-eyed peas.						
Cucumber slices, 1/8 in. thick (large, 2 1/8-in. diam.; small, 1 3/4-in. diam.):						
With peel	6 large or 8 small	28	95	5	Trace	Trace
Without peel	6 1/2 large or 9 small pieces	28	96	5	Trace	Trace
Dandelion greens, cooked, drained	1 c	105	90	35	2	1
Endive, curly (including escarole), raw, small pieces	1 c	50	93	10	1	Trace
Kale, cooked, drained:						
From raw (leaves without stems and midribs)	1 c	110	88	45	5	1
From frozen (leaf style)	1 c	130	91	40	4	1
Lettuce, raw:						
Butter head, as Boston types:						
Head, 5-in. diam.	1	220[63]	95	25	2	Trace
Leaves	1 outer, 2 inner, or 3 heart leaves	15	95	Trace	Trace	Trace
Crisp head, as iceberg:						
Head, 6-in. diam.	1	567[64]	96	70	5	1
Wedge, 1/4 of head	1	135	96	20	1	Trace
Pieces, chopped or shredded	1 c	55	96	5	Trace	Trace
Loose leaf (bunching varieties including romaine), chopped or shredded pieced	1 c	55	94	10	1	Trace
Mushrooms, raw, sliced, or chopped	1 c	70	90	20	2	Trace
Mustard greens, without stems and midribs, cooked, drained	1 c	140	93	30	3	1
Okra pods, 3 by 5/8 in., cooked	10	106	91	30	2	Trace
Onions:						
Mature:						
Raw:						
Chopped	1 c	170	89	65	3	Trace
Sliced	1 c	115	89	45	2	Trace
Cooked (whole or sliced) drained	1 c	210	92	60	3	Trace
Young green, bulb (3/8-in. diam.) and white portion of top	6 onions	30	88	15	Trace	Trace
Parsley, raw, chopped	1 T	4	85	Trace	Trace	Trace
Parsnips, cooked (diced or 2-in. lengths)	1 c	155	82	100	2	1

NUTRIENTS IN INDICATED QUANTITY

FATTY ACIDS			Carbohydrate (g)	Calcium (mg)	Phosphorus (mg)	Iron (mg)	Potassium (mg)	Vitamin A Value (IU)	Vitamin B1 (mg)	Vitamin B2 (mg)	Niacin (mg)	Vitamin C (mg)
Saturated (Total) (g)	Unsaturated Oleic (g)	Unsaturated Linoleic (g)										
—	—	—	27	4	121	1.0	291	440[62]	0.18	0.10	2.1	9
—	—	—	31	5	120	1.3	304	580[62]	0.15	0.10	2.5	8
—	—	—	51	8	143	1.5	248	840[62]	0.08	0.13	2.6	13
—	—	—	43	6	153	1.1	204	740[62]	0.06	0.13	2.3	11
—	—	—	33	8	81	0.8	160	580[62]	0.05	0.08	1.5	7
—	—	—	1	7	8	0.3	45	70	0.01	0.01	0.1	3
—	—	—	1	5	5	0.1	45	Trace	0.01	0.01	0.1	3
—	—	—	7	147	44	1.9	244	12,290	0.14	0.17	—	19
—	—	—	2	41	27	0.9	147	1,650	0.04	0.07	0.3	5
—	—	—	7	206	64	1.8	243	9,130	0.11	0.20	1.8	102
—	—	—	7	157	62	1.3	251	10,660	0.08	0.20	0.9	49
—	—	—	4	57	42	3.3	430	1,580	0.10	0.10	0.5	13
—	—	—	Trace	5	4	0.3	40	150	0.01	0.01	Trace	1
—	—	—	16	108	118	2.7	943	1,780	0.32	0.32	1.6	32
—	—	—	4	27	30	0.7	236	450	0.08	0.08	0.4	8
—	—	—	2	11	12	0.3	96	180	0.03	0.03	0.2	3
—	—	—	2	37	14	0.8	145	1,050	0.03	0.04	0.2	10
—	—	—	3	4	81	0.6	290	Trace	0.07	0.32	2.9	2
—	—	—	6	193	45	2.5	308	8,120	0.11	0.20	0.8	67
—	—	—	6	98	43	0.5	184	520	0.14	0.19	1.0	21
—	—	—	15	46	61	0.9	267	Trace[65]	0.05	0.07	0.3	17
—	—	—	10	31	41	0.6	181	Trace[65]	0.03	0.05	0.2	12
—	—	—	14	50	61	0.8	231	Trace[65]	0.06	0.06	0.4	15
—	—	—	3	12	12	0.2	69	Trace	0.02	0.01	0.1	8
—	—	—	Trace	7	2	0.2	25	300	Trace	0.01	Trace	6
—	—	—	23	70	96	0.9	587	50	0.11	0.12	0.2	16

FOOD	Approximate Measures. Units. or Weight	Weight (g)	Water (%)	Food Energy (C)	Protein (g)	Fat (g)
Peas, green:						
Canned:						
Whole, drained solids	1 c	170	77	150	8	1
Strained (baby food)	1 oz (1¾–2 T)	28	86	15	1	Trace
Frozen, cooked, drained	1 c	160	82	110	8	Trace
Peppers, hot, red, without seeds, dried (ground chili powder, added seasonings)	1 t	2	9	5	Trace	Trace
Peppers, sweet (about 5 per pound, whole), stem and seeds removed:						
Raw	1 pod	74	93	15	1	Trace
Cooked, boiled, drained	1 pod	73	95	15	1	Trace
Potatoes, cooked:						
Baked, peeled after baking (about 2 per pound, raw)	1	156	75	145	4	Trace
Boiled (about 3 per pound, raw):						
Peeled after boiling	1	137	80	105	3	Trace
Peeled before boiling	1	135	83	90	3	Trace
French fries, 2 to 3½ in. long:						
Prepared from raw	10	50	45	135	2	7
Frozen, oven heated	10	50	53	110	2	4
Hashed brown, prepared from frozen	1 c	155	56	345	3	18
Mashed, prepared from—						
Raw:						
Milk added	1 c	210	83	135	4	2
Milk and butter added	1 c	210	80	195	4	9
Dehydrated flakes (without milk), water, milk, butter, and salt added	1 c	210	79	195	4	7
Potato chips, 1¾ by 2½ in. oval cross section	10	20	2	115	1	8
Potato salad, made with cooked salad dressing	1 c	250	76	250	7	7
Pumpkin, canned	1 c	245	90	80	2	1
Radishes, raw (prepackaged) stem ends, rootlets cut off	4	18	95	5	Trace	Trace
Sauerkraut, canned, solids, and liquid	1 c	235	93	40	2	Trace
Southern peas. See Black-eyed peas.						
Spinach:						
Raw, chopped	1 c	55	91	15	2	Trace
Canned, drained solids	1 c	205	91	50	6	1
Cooked, drained:						
From raw	1 c	180	92	40	5	1
From frozen:						
Chopped	1 c	205	92	45	6	1
Leaf	1 c	190	92	45	6	1
Squash, cooked:						
Summer (all varieties), diced, drained	1 c	210	96	30	2	Trace
Winter (all varieties), baked, mashed	1 c	205	81	130	4	1

NUTRIENTS IN INDICATED QUANTITY

Saturated (Total) (g)	Unsaturated Oleic (g)	Unsaturated Linoleic (g)	Carbohydrate (g)	Calcium (mg)	Phosphorus (mg)	Iron (mg)	Potassium (mg)	Vitamin A Value (IU)	Vitamin B1 (mg)	Vitamin B2 (mg)	Niacin (mg)	Vitamin C (mg)
							FATTY ACIDS header					
—	—	—	29	44	129	3.2	163	1,170	0.15	0.10	1.4	14
—	—	—	3	3	18	0.3	28	140	0.02	0.03	0.3	3
—	—	—	19	30	138	3.0	216	960	0.43	0.14	2.7	21
—	—	—	1	5	4	0.3	20	1,300	Trace	0.02	0.2	Trace
—	—	—	4	7	16	0.5	157	310	0.06	0.06	0.4	94
—	—	—	3	7	12	0.4	109	310	0.05	0.05	0.4	70
—	—	—	33	14	101	1.1	782	Trace	0.15	0.07	2.7	31
—	—	—	23	10	72	0.8	556	Trace	0.12	0.05	2.0	22
—	—	—	20	8	57	0.7	385	Trace	0.12	0.05	1.6	22
1.7	1.2	3.3	18	8	56	0.7	427	Trace	0.07	0.04	1.6	11
1.1	.8	2.1	17	5	43	0.9	326	Trace	0.07	0.01	1.3	11
4.6	3.2	9.0	45	28	78	1.9	439	Trace	0.11	0.03	1.6	12
0.7	0.4	Trace	27	50	103	0.8	548	40	0.17	0.11	2.1	21
5.6	2.3	0.2	26	50	101	0.8	525	360	0.17	0.11	2.1	19
3.6	2.1	0.2	30	65	99	0.6	601	270	0.08	0.08	1.9	11
2.1	1.4	4.0	10	8	28	0.4	226	Trace	0.04	0.01	1.0	3
2.0	2.7	1.3	41	80	160	1.5	798	350	0.20	0.18	2.8	28
—	—	—	19	61	64	1.0	588	15,680	0.07	0.12	1.5	12
—	—	—	1	5	6	0.2	58	Trace	0.01	0.01	0.1	5
—	—	—	9	85	42	1.2	329	120	0.07	0.09	0.5	33
—	—	—	2	51	28	1.7	259	4,460	0.06	0.11	0.3	28
—	—	—	7	242	53	5.3	513	16,400	0.04	0.25	0.6	29
—	—	—	6	167	68	4.0	583	14,580	0.13	0.25	0.9	50
—	—	—	8	232	90	4.3	683	16,200	0.14	0.31	0.8	39
—	—	—	7	200	84	4.8	688	15,390	0.15	0.27	1.0	53
—	—	—	7	53	53	0.8	296	820	0.11	0.17	1.7	21
—	—	—	32	57	98	1.6	945	8,610	0.10	0.27	1.4	27

FOOD	Approximate Measures, Units, or Weight	Weight (g)	Water (%)	Food Energy (C)	Protein (g)	Fat (g)
Sweet potatoes:						
Candied, 2½ × 2 in. piece	1 piece	105	60	175	1	3
Canned						
Solid pack (mashed)	1 c	255	72	275	5	1
Vacuum pack, 2¾ × 1 in. piece	1 piece	40	72	45	1	Trace
Cooked (raw, 5 × 2 in.; about 2½ per pound):						
Baked in skin, peeled	1	114	64	160	2	1
Boiled in skin, peeled	1	151	71	170	3	1
Tomatoes:						
Raw, 2⅗-in. diam. (3 per 12-oz package)	1	135⁶⁶	94	25	1	Trace
Canned, solids and liquid	1 c	241	94	50	2	Trace
Tomato catsup	1 c	273	69	290	5	1
	1 T	15	69	15	Trace	Trace
Tomato juice, canned:						
Cup	1 c	243	94	45	2	Trace
Glass	6 fl oz	182	94	35	2	Trace
Turnips, cooked, diced	1 c	155	94	35	1	Trace
Turnip greens, cooked, drained:						
From raw (leaves and stems)	1 c	145	94	30	3	Trace
From frozen (chopped)	1 c	165	93	40	4	Trace
Vegetables, mixed, frozen, cooked	1 c	182	83	115	6	1
Miscellaneous items						
Baking powders for home use:						
Sodium aluminum sulfate:						
With monocalcium phosphate monohydrate	1 t	3.0	2	5	Trace	Trace
With monocalcium phosphate monohydrate, calcium sulfate	1 t	2.9	1	5	Trace	Trace
Straight phosphate	1 t	3.8	2	5	Trace	Trace
Low sodium	1 t	4.3	2	5	Trace	Trace
Barbecue sauce	1 c	250	81	230	4	17
Beverages, alcoholic:						
Beer	12 fl oz	360	92	150	1	0
Gin, rum, vodka, whisky:						
80 proof	1½-fl oz (jigger)	42	67	95	—	—
86 proof	1½-fl oz (jigger)	42	64	105	—	—
90 proof	1½-fl oz (jigger)	42	62	110	—	—
Wines:						
Dessert	3½ fl oz	103	77	140	Trace	0
Table	3½ fl oz	102	86	85	Trace	0
Beverages, carbonated, sweetened, nonalcoholic:						
Carbonated water	12 fl oz	366	92	115	0	0
Cola type	12 fl oz	369	90	145	0	0
Fruit-flavored sodas and Tom Collins mixer	12 fl oz	372	88	170	0	0

| FATTY ACIDS | | | | | | | | | | | | |
Saturated (Total) (g)	Unsaturated Oleic (g)	Unsaturated Linoleic (g)	Carbohydrate (g)	Calcium (mg)	Phosphorus (mg)	Iron (mg)	Potassium (mg)	Vitamin A Value (IU)	Vitamin B1 (mg)	Vitamin B2 (mg)	Niacin (mg)	Vitamin C (mg)
2.0	0.8	0.1	36	39	45	0.9	200	6,620	0.06	0.04	0.4	11
—	—	—	63	64	105	2.0	510	19,890	0.13	0.10	1.5	36
—	—	—	10	10	16	0.3	80	3,120	0.02	0.02	0.2	6
—	—	—	37	46	66	1.0	342	9,230	0.10	0.08	0.8	25
—	—	—	40	48	71	1.1	367	11,940	0.14	0.09	0.9	26
—	—	—	6	16	33	0.6	300	1,110	0.07	0.05	0.9	28[67]
—	—	—	10	14[68]	46	1.2	523	2,170	0.12	0.07	1.7	41
—	—	—	69	60	137	2.2	991	3,820	0.25	0.19	4.4	41
—	—	—	4	3	8	0.1	54	210	0.01	0.01	0.2	2
—	—	—	10	17	44	2.2	552	1,940	0.12	0.07	1.0	39
—	—	—	8	13	33	1.6	413	1,460	0.09	0.05	1.5	29
—	—	—	8	54	37	0.6	291	Trace	0.06	0.08	0.5	34
—	—	—	5	252	49	1.5	—	8,270	0.15	0.33	0.7	68
—	—	—	6	195	64	2.6	246	11,390	0.08	0.15	0.7	31
—	—	—	24	46	115	2.4	348	9,010	0.22	0.13	2.0	15
0	0	0	1	58	87	—	5	0	0	0	0	0
0	0	0	1	183	45	—	—	0	0	0	0	0
0	0	0	1	239	359	—	6	0	0	0	0	0
0	0	0	2	207	314	—	471	0	0	0	0	0
2.2	4.3	10.0	20	53	50	2.0	435	900	0.03	0.03	0.8	13
0	0	0	14	18	108	Trace	90	—	0.01	0.11	2.2	—
0	0	0	Trace	—	—	—	1	—	—	—	—	—
0	0	0	Trace	—	—	—	1	—	—	—	—	—
0	0	0	Trace	—	—	—	1	—	—	—	—	—
0	0	0	8	8	—	—	77	—	0.01	0.02	0.2	—
0	0	0	4	9	10	0.4	94	—	Trace	0.01	0.1	—
0	0	0	29	—	—	—	—	0	0	0	0	0
0	0	0	37	—	—	—	—	0	0	0	0	0
0	0	0	45	—	—	—	—	0	0	0	0	0

FOOD	Approximate Measures, Units, or Weight	Weight (g)	Water (%)	Food Energy (C)	Protein (g)	Fat (g)
Ginger ale	12 fl oz	366	92	115	0	0
Root beer	12 fl oz	370	90	150	0	0
Chili powder. See Peppers, hot, red.						
Chocolate:						
Bitter or baking	1 oz	28	2	145	3	15
Semisweet, see Candy: Chocolate.						
Gelatin, dry	7 g	7	13	25	6	Trace
Gelatin dessert prepared with gelatin dessert						
powder and water	1 c	240	84	140	4	0
Mustard, prepared, yellow	1 t or individual serving pouch or cup	5	80	5	Trace	Trace
Olives, pickled, canned:						
Green:	4 medium, 3 extra large, or 2 giant	16[69]	78	15	Trace	2
Ripe, Mission	3 small or 2 large	10[69]	73	15	Trace	2
Pickles, cucumber:						
Dill, medium, whole, 3¾ in. long, 1¼-in. diam.	1 pickle	65	93	5	Trace	Trace
Fresh pack, slices 1½-in. diam., ¼ in. thick	2 slices	15	79	10	Trace	Trace
Sweet, gherkin, small, whole, about 2½ in. long, ¾-in. diam.	1 pickle	15	61	20	Trace	Trace
Relish, finely chopped, sweet	1 T	15	63	20	Trace	Trace
Popcorn. See items 476–478.						
Popsicle	3 fl oz	95	80	70	0	0
Soups:						
Canned, condensed:						
Prepared with equal volume of milk:						
Cream of Chicken	1 c	245	85	180	7	10
Cream of mushroom	1 c	245	83	215	7	14
Tomato	1 c	250	84	175	7	7
Prepared with equal volume of water:						
Bean with pork	1 c	250	84	170	8	6
Beef broth, bouillon, consommé	1 c	240	96	30	5	0
Beef noodle	1 c	240	93	65	4	3
Clam chowder, Manhattan type (with tomatoes, without milk)	1 c	245	92	80	2	3
Cream of chicken	1 c	240	92	95	3	6
Cream of mushroom	1 c	240	90	135	2	10
Minestrone	1 c	245	90	105	5	3
Split pea	1 c	245	85	145	9	3
Tomato	1 c	245	91	90	2	3
Vegetable beef	1 c	245	92	80	5	2
Vegetarian	1 c	245	92	80	2	2

NUTRIENTS IN INDICATED QUANTITY

FATTY ACIDS			Carbohydrate (g)	Calcium (mg)	Phosphorus (mg)	Iron (mg)	Potassium (mg)	Vitamin A Value (IU)	Vitamin B1 (mg)	Vitamin B2 (mg)	Niacin (mg)	Vitamin C (mg)
Saturated (Total) (g)	Unsaturated Oleic (g)	Unsaturated Linoleic (g)										
0	0	0	29	—	—	—	0	0	0	0	0	0
0	0	0	39	—	—	—	0	0	0	0	0	0
8.9	4.9	0.4	8	22	109	1.9	235	20	0.01	0.07	0.4	0
0	0	0	0	—	—	—	—	—	—	—	—	—
0	0	0	34	—	—	—	—	—	—	—	—	—
—	—	—	Trace	4	4	0.1	7	—	—	—	—	—
0.2	1.2	0.1	Trace	8	2	0.2	7	40	—	—	—	—
0.2	1.2	0.1	Trace	9	1	0.1	2	10	Trace	Trace	—	—
—	—	—	1	17	14	0.7	130	70	Trace	0.01	Trace	4
—	—	—	3	5	4	0.3	—	20	Trace	Trace	Trace	1
—	—	—	5	2	2	0.2	—	10	Trace	Trace	Trace	1
—	—	—	5	3	2	0.1	—	—	—	—	—	—
0	0	0	18	0	—	Trace	—	0	0	0	0	0
4.2	3.6	1.3	15	172	152	0.5	260	610	0.05	0.27	0.7	2
5.4	2.9	4.6	16	191	169	0.5	279	250	0.05	0.34	0.7	1
3.4	1.7	1.0	23	168	155	0.8	418	1,200	0.10	0.25	1.3	15
1.2	1.8	2.4	22	63	128	2.3	395	650	0.13	0.08	1.0	3
0	0	0	3	Trace	31	0.5	130	Trace	Trace	0.02	1.2	—
0.6	0.7	0.8	7	7	48	1.0	77	50	0.05	0.07	1.0	Trace
0.5	0.4	1.3	12	34	47	1.0	184	880	0.02	0.02	1.0	—
1.6	2.3	1.1	8	24	34	0.5	79	410	0.02	0.05	0.5	Trace
2.6	1.7	4.5	10	41	50	0.5	98	70	0.02	0.12	0.7	Trace
0.7	0.9	1.3	14	37	59	1.0	314	2,350	0.07	0.05	1.0	—
1.1	1.2	0.4	21	29	149	1.5	270	440	0.25	0.15	1.5	1
0.5	0.5	1.0	16	15	34	0.7	230	1,000	0.05	0.05	1.2	12
—	—	—	10	12	49	0.7	162	2,700	0.05	0.05	1.0	—
—	—	—	13	20	39	1.0	172	2,940	0.05	0.05	1.0	—

FOOD	Approximate Measures, Units, or Weight	Weight (g)	Water (%)	Food Energy (C)	Protein (g)	Fat (g)
Dehydrated:						
Bouillon cube, ½ in.	1 cube	4	4	5	1	Trace
Mixes:						
Unprepared:						
Onion	1½ oz	43	3	150	6	5
Prepared with water:						
Chicken noodle	1 c	240	95	55	2	1
Onion	1 c	240	96	35	1	1
Tomato vegetable with noodles	1 c	240	93	65	1	1
Vinegar, cider	1 T	15	94	Trace	Trace	0
White sauce, medium, with enriched flour	1 c	250	73	405	10	31
Yeast:						
Baker's dry, active	1 package	7	5	20	3	Trace
Brewer's, dry	1 T	8	5	25	3	Trace

[1] Vitamin A value is largely from β-carotene used for coloring. Riboflavin value for powdered creamers apply to products with added riboflavin.

[2] Applies to product without added vitamin A. With added vitamin A, value is 500 IU.

[3] Applies to product without added vitamin A.

[4] Applies to product with added vitamin A. Without added vitamin A, value is 20 IU.

[5] Yields 1 qt of fluid milk when reconstituted according to package directions.

[6] Applies to product with added vitamin A.

[7] Weight applies to product with label claim of 1⅓ cups equal 3.2 oz.

[8] Applies to products made from thick shake mixes with no added ice cream. Products made from milk shake mixes are higher in fat and usually contain added ice cream.

[9] Content of fat, vitamin A, and carbohydrate varies. Consult the label when precise values are needed for special diets.

[10] Applies to product made with milk containing no added vitamin A.

[11] Based on year-round average.

[12] Based on average vitamin A content of fortified margarine. Federal specifications for fortified margarine require a minimum of 15,000 IU of vitamin A per pound.

[13] Fatty acid values apply to product made with regular margarine.

[14] Dipped in egg, milk or water, and bread crumbs; fried in vegetable shortening.

[15] If bones are discarded, value for calcium will be greatly reduced.

[16] Dipped in egg, bread crumbs, and flour or batter.

[17] Prepared with tuna, celery, salad dressing (mayonnaise type), pickle, onion, and egg.

[18] Outer layer of fat on the cut removed to within approximately ½ in. of the lean. Deposits of fat within the cut not removed.

[19] Crust made with vegetable shortening and enriched flour.

[20] Regular margarine used.

[21] Value varies widely.

[22] About one-fourth of the outer layer of fat on the cut removed. Deposits of fat within the cut not removed.

[23] Vegetable shortening used.

[24] Also applies to pasteurized apple cider.

[25] Applies to product without added ascorbic acid. For value of product with added ascorbic acid, refer to label.

[26] Based on product with label claim of 45% of U.S. RDA in 6 fl oz.

[27] Based on product with label claim of 100% of U.S. RDA in 6 fl oz.

FATTY ACIDS Saturated (Total) (g)	Unsaturated Oleic (g)	Unsaturated Linoleic (g)	Carbohydrate (g)	Calcium (mg)	Phosphorus (mg)	Iron (mg)	Potassium (mg)	Vitamin A Value (IU)	Vitamin B1 (mg)	Vitamin B2 (mg)	Niacin (mg)	Vitamin C (mg)
—	—	—	Trace	—	—	—	4	—	—	—	—	—
1.1	2.3	1.0	23	42	49	0.6	238	30	0.05	0.03	0.3	6
—	—	—	8	7	19	0.2	19	50	0.07	0.05	0.5	Trace
—	—	—	6	10	12	0.2	58	Trace	Trace	Trace	Trace	2
—	—	—	12	7	19	0.2	29	480	0.05	0.02	0.5	5
0	0	0	1	1	1	0.1	15	—	—	—	—	—
19.3	7.8	0.8	22	288	233	0.5	348	1,150	0.12	0.43	0.7	2
—	—	—	3	3	90	1.1	140	Trace	0.16	0.38	2.6	Trace
—	—	—	3	17[70]	140	1.4	152	Trace	1.25	0.34	3.0	Trace

[28] Weight includes peel and membranes between sections. Without these parts, the weight of the edible portion is 123 g for pink or red grapefruit and 118 g for white.

[29] For white-fleshed varieties, value is about 20 IU per cup; for red-fleshed varieties, 1,080 IU.

[30] Weight includes seeds. Without seeds, weight of the edible portion is 57 g.

[31] Applies to product without added ascorbic acid. With added ascorbic acid, based on claim that 6 fl oz of reconstituted juice contain 45% or 50% of the U.S. RDA, value is 108 or 120 mg for a 6-fl-oz can and 36 or 40 mg for 1 c of diluted juice.

[32] For products with added thiamin and riboflavin but without added ascorbic acid, values in milligrams would be 0.60 for thiamin, 0.80 for riboflavin, and a trace for ascorbic acid. For products with only ascorbic acid added, value varies with the brand. Consult the label.

[33] Weight includes rind. Without rind, the weight of the edible portion is 272 g for cantaloupe and 149 g for honeydew.

[34] Represents yellow-fleshed varieties. For white-fleshed varieties, value is 50 IU for 1 peach and 90 IU for 1 c of slices.

[35] Value represents products with added ascorbic acid. For products without added ascorbic acid, the values are highly variable; e.g., 10–25 mg for a 10-oz container, and 15–35 mg for 1 c.

[36] Weight includes pits. After removal of the pits, the weight of the edible portion is 258 g for a cup and 133 g for a portion, 43 g for uncooked prunes, and 213 g for cooked prunes.

[37] Weight includes rind and seeds. Without rind and seeds, weight of the edible portion is 426 g.

[38] Made with vegetable shortening.

[39] Applies to product made with white cornmeal. With yellow cornmeal, value is 30 IU.

[40] Applies to white varieties. For yellow varieties, value is 150 IU.

[41] Applies to products that do not contain disodium phosphate. If disodium phosphate is an ingredient, value is 162 mg.

[42] Value may range from less than 1 mg to about 8 mg, depending on the brand. Consult the label.

[43] Applies to product with added nutrient. Without added nutrient, value is trace.

[44] Value varies with the brand. Consult the label.

[45] Applies to product with added nutrient. Without added nutrient, value is trace.

[46] Except for angel food cake, cakes were made from mixes containing vegetable shortening; icings made from butter.

[47] Except for sponge cake, vegetable shortening used for cake portion; butter, for icing. If

butter or margarine used for cake portion, vitamin A values are higher.

[48] Applies to product made with a sodium-aluminum-sulfate-type baking powder. With a low-sodium baking powder containing potassium, value would be about twice the amount shown.

[49] Equal weights of flour, sugar, eggs, and vegetable shortening.

[50] Products are commercial unless otherwise specified.

[51] Made with enriched flour and vegetable shortening except for macaroons, which do not contain flour or shortening.

[52] Icing made with butter.

[53] Applies to yellow varieties; white varieties contain only a trace.

[54] Contains vegetable shortening and butter.

[55] Made with corn oil.

[56] Made with regular margarine.

[57] Applies to product made with yellow cornmeal.

[58] Made with enriched degermed cornmeal and enriched flour.

[59] Product may or may not be enriched with riboflavin. Consult the label.

[60] Value varies with the brand. Consult the label.

[61] Weight includes cob. Without cob, weight is 77 g for a raw ear and 126 g for a frozen ear.

[62] Based on yellow varieties. For white varieties, value is trace.

[63] Weight includes refuse of outer leaves and core. Without these parts, weight is 163 g.

[64] Weight includes core. Without core, weight is 539 g.

[65] Value based on white-fleshed varieties. For yellow-fleshed varieties, value is 70 IU for chopped raw onions, 50 IU for sliced raw onions.

[66] Weight includes cores and stem ends. Without these parts, weight is 123 g.

[67] Based on year-round average. For tomatoes marketed from November through May, value is about 12 mg; from June through October, 21 mg.

[68] Applies to product without calcium salts added. Value for products with calcium salts added may be as much as 63 mg.

[69] Weight includes pits. Without pits, weight is 13 g for green olives and 9 g for Mission ripe olives.

[70] Value may vary from 6 to 60 mg.

Source: Home & Garden Bulletin No. 72, Government Printing Office, Washington, D.C.